# Keto Diet - The Complete Guide

*Clarity, Simply and Easy Getting Started Guide for Lose Weight, Health and Fat Burn with Meal Plan and Low Carb Recipes for Ketogenic Diet in Busy People*

# Table of Contents

# Introduction

A good diet is extremely important not just to have a nice body, but most importantly to be healthy. Often times, a healthy body translates to a healthy mind, and in this book, you will not only learn everything about the ketogenic diet, but you will also discover how it can have a positive impact on your lifestyle as well.

We understand how difficult it can be for people to lose fat and get back in shape, especially after stressful times and events. You are running around all day trying to provide for your family and there is not too much time left to focus on good eating habits. Even though this is certainly true, it does not mean that you should give up on your health. There are a lot of methods that allow the everyday busy person to eat healthily and take care of their body, even if they do not have a lot of spare time.

This is why we decided to create this book. After helping thousands of people lose belly fat and gain a better lifestyle, we had to write down what we know, so that everyone can benefit from our knowledge. The ketogenic diet is a great tool to get in shape efficiently, while taking care of your body and without stressing out about dieting. It is a nutritional regiment that is easy to follow and that a lot of people, both men and women, have found beneficial.

Inside this book, we are going to reveal you everything there is to know about ketogenic diet, providing you with all the tools and strategies to make it work properly. The secret to losing weight is being able to keep it off when the "diet" ends. We do not believe in the concept of dieting and believe that the ketogenic diet can be a lifestyle. If you approach it with the same mindset, you can be sure you will have a lot of success and see results very fast!

There are hundreds of books on this topic, so thank you for choosing this one. Now let's dive into the topic and get healthier together!

# Chapter 1: It Starts with Your Mind

"I'll start my diet on Monday!" How many times have we said this sentence or heard it. But that Monday for some people never comes or lasts a day. Here come the failures or the odious yo-yo effect, which often brings with it a lot of dissatisfaction in addition to the anti-aesthetic effect of stretch marks.

It's true that keeping the weight is not easy, especially when the finances and sources of income are so low that many people are having a hard time keeping up with their basic needs, even with their food. This is considering that while the vegetables are paid by weight, the so-called junk food offers bargain prices.

Another element that certainly does not make in favor of diets is the time factor. In a company that has always counted the minutes, you prefer a hypercaloric sandwich than ordering a healthy slice of steamed meat ... and when you come back home late from work, the temptation of ready-made food is strong!

But it is equally true that diet is, first of all, a matter of the right mindset. If we enter the right mindset, there are no tight finances or tight deadlines.

**Tell Me Why You Eat**

First, we must ask ourselves how much and what we eat for hunger and for other reasons. Often, anger, sadness, insecurity, or boredom makes us open the fridge to unplug at least for that period of time. It is the theory of compensation. It is the simplest, immediate, and most usable way to console yourself - often with sweet or otherwise high-calorie foods - from something in our life that we do not like or do not accept. This can result in more additional problems aside from psychological consequences because it can add more unnecessary weight which can become your physical problem.

A short assessment of why we are swallowing food can help us understand what problem we need to solve or focus on what we would like to improve in our lives, and at the same time, block a sense of hunger that comes from the mind and not the stomach.

**Psychological Tricks in the Kitchen**

To give help to our willpower, we can put simple tricks into practice:

We know that the eye wants its part. And it is equally known that every taste is also involved in nutrition. We are not inclined to eat a dish with unpleasant odor even if the taste is good. In the same way, a not well-presented dish sends negative messages to the brain. It is no coincidence that the chefs' skills are also a factor in the presentation of the dishes. The problem of portion reductions is often because of the lack of contents present in the dish. We must, therefore, circumvent the obstacle such as putting out 80 grams of pasta in a smaller-sized dish instead of a regular sized plate. This can trick us to think that were already consuming a large amount of food when we're actually not.

"I can resist anything but temptation," said Oscar Wilde, which when translated means learning to make a reasoned expense. Avoid keeping snacks, chocolates, junk food or anything that moves you away from the right path. At the same time, do not forget to buy healthy snacks, which can also easily be carried out or in the office such as an apple.

Finally, realistic goals must be set. Thinking of doing lightning diets or losing an exaggerated number of pounds would be detrimental to health, and in many cases, often unattainable. This will only result to failures and frustrations which can lead to giving up. It is best to follow the advice of the professionals and always set realistic steps so that motivation wouldn't be lost and you can keep continuing having proper nutrition.

Here are the five tips to adopt the right psychology to lose weight:

**RECOGNIZE THAT YOU CAN**

Let's start by realizing that you can reach your ideal body unless you suffer from a disease that does not allow you to lose weight. Recognize that you can do it, that you have no real impediment to achieving the right weight. Look around and look for people in your same situation who maintained their weight or who have lost excess weight in a healthy and lasting way.

## IMPOSE YOUR WILL TO YOUR STOMACH

Make yourself aware that it is the stomach that decides. The stomach chooses when it is hungry when it is full and not you. Listen and respect the signals that your body is giving you. How much time has passed since you heard your stomach make a strange noise due to hunger? If too much time has passed, rediscover it. How much time has passed since you got up from the table still with a sense of lightness and full of energy?

## BE POSITIVE

But not in the sense that you "hope" that everything goes well and you put bandages on your eyes when difficulties appear. I mean talk positively, encourage yourself, correct what you want, and erase what you no longer desire. Do not say what you do not want, but focus on what you desire to achieve. Talk to the present about what you want to be, do, and believe.

## DO NOT LISTEN TO YOUR MIND

Think that the taste of something must always be associated with true hunger. If there is no real hunger, then the will to eat something tasty will wait patiently. Otherwise, you can satisfy your hunger with very small treats and enjoy them to the last one.

We all know that there are foods we are supposed to eat to be healthy and others that is better to stay away from. The news is constantly flooded by articles that tell us what we can and what we cannot consume. And if that is not enough, many of these messages sent to the population today are transmitted through media, internet, and often by professionals in the food sector as well.

So, it is understandable to be lost in a world that, on one hand, does not lose a second to put under the nose and before the eyes, all kinds of desserts and, on the other hand, informs us about how they hurt and have a negative effect on our health.

A phrase that I often heard from people as a strategy to resist the temptations is the following:

> "Remember, 10 seconds in the mouth and then 10 years in the belly."

And so it is that in people, especially those who embark on a path of weight loss, conflicting feelings are created. On one side, there is the desire and the pleasure of consuming food such as a slice of chocolate cake, while, on the other, there is the sense of failure and guilt once the dessert has been eaten.

## Prohibited Foods, Self-Control, and Guilt: The Recipe for Catastrophe

The desire for "forbidden" foods leads to the strain on our self-control by placing us in front of a "late-cost dilemma". Eating that cake today means I could enjoy the flavor and social context in which consumption takes place (immediate effect), but tomorrow, I will pay the consequences of my gesture with a little extra fat (delayed effect).

Even in public health circles, there is a strong conviction that to establish a certain degree of guilt towards unhealthy types of foods leads people to limit themselves in the consumption of those foods, pushing them towards healthier and better choices. This is a strategy that has been around for quite some time, and a lot of people have swayed towards it.

Unfortunately, the effects of guilt were not the desired ones.

In fact, we should consider that even the sense of guilt produces two different realities. The reality before doing the undesirable act of consuming is a positive sense of guilt that leads us to reflect on what we want to do and, that, therefore, could have positive implications in guiding our choices. The sense of guilt that is born and continues after having consumed our forbidden slice of chocolate cake is a negative sense of guilt that hardly ever leads to positive implications, and that is the more frequent of the two.

In most cases, the motivational reason we consume foods not provided by our nutritional plan is much stronger than the sense of guilt that is perceived beforehand. Therefore, guilt does not stop us from yielding to temptation. Often, we do not even have the time to implement rational corrective actions because the impulse to grab and put food in the mouth is too rapid. Once the consumption is completed, the sense of guilt is amplified, bringing with it self-criticism, loss of control, and loss of self-esteem.

A catastrophe-effect – driven by the sense of a lack of self-discipline – is triggered. For those people who are on a diet, the sense of guilt that follows a small cheat in the diet turns into a point of no return, a full loss of control without the possibility of remedy, and in your head, you hear that voice that says, "Great, now the damage is done, do whatever you want."

Some studies have compared groups of people who perceive "forbidden" foods as gratification/reward/celebration or as gimmicks/reasons for feeling guilty after observing how these feelings and perceptions about food affect their body weight and habit food.

It showed that the sense of guilt does not push people to have better eating habits and does not lead to better weight control over the short term or the long term. On the contrary, these subjects tend to maintain or increase their weight over time and have a tendency toward disordered eating that is pervaded by periods of restriction and binge eating. A further negative consequence of this guilt mentality is the increasingly low self-esteem they feel and the lack of confidence in their ability to improve as a person.

The people who, instead, perceive food that is usually considered "forbidden" as a food destined for moments of happiness and celebration have shown a greater awareness of food and make better choices in their usual diet. This perception has consequently led to a reduction in weight (if necessary) or to the maintenance of weight in both the short- and long-term. These people have better self-control as well because they are not driven by a compelling impulse, which is generated by food deprivation.

## Freedom and Flexibility: The Recipe for Long-Term Weight Loss

To associate "cheat meals" with moments of happiness and celebration has been related to greater results and better maintenance over time.

According to Fredrickson's "broaden-and-build" theory, a positive state of mind is a resource that makes issues like "self-control problems" simpler to deal with. This goes back to positive thinking and the idea that we attract what we focus on. Have you ever had the feeling that everything goes wrong when you are in a bad mood? Well, the same goes for dieting. If you keep thinking and focusing on the fact that you are giving up your favorite food, it will be difficult to keep at it. On the other hand, by constantly reminding why you are doing it and what is the goal you are trying to achieve, you will be in a much better position. It is not just philosophy, as you will see in the following pages. There have been many research studies on this topic.

Studies have shown that a positive attitude increases the ability to resist the temptation to eat "unhealthy foods." To conclude this discussion, a sense of guilt does not lead to positive adaptations. Giving people the knowledge about what they consume through programs, inputs, and campaigns on healthy eating do not lead to real improvement.

The pleasure of eating a good meal in a context of joy, serenity, gratification, or celebration without experiencing a sense of guilt but rather with awareness, even if it is made up of "forbidden" foods may lead to better management of your diet in the long term.

Therefore, it is appropriate to develop your mindset towards an easier, less rigid attitude. Some extra gratification inserted into your diet, in a planned and conscious way, will lead to better and longer-lasting result while reducing stress caused by excessive limitations.

## Use Cheat Meals for Assured Success

We have understood that being too rigid in food choices and depriving ourselves of anything that could potentially alienate us from our physical fitness goal is not the best solution. What to do then?

Follow the advice of Oscar Wilde to the letter: "The only way to get rid of a temptation is to yield to it. Resist it, and your soul grows sick with longing...." Surely, resisting would only serve to get us away from our goals, so here is an alternate path to follow.

Plan one or more weekly "cheat" meals within your diet plan (the number will depend on the objective, the condition of your body, etc.) to gratify yourself and without any sense of guilt.

If, in the same week, there were more occasions, adjust the pre- and post-cheat-meals to minimize the effects of those extra calories.

And what do you do if there are unshakable reasons that make an entire box of cookies desirable? Rule number 1: Learn to stop before starting. Procrastinate and let the tide settle, because stopping after biting the first cookie will be very, very difficult. Trust me, I have been there and have done it.

The first thing to understand is that when this happens, there is something that does not work in the way of reacting to emotion or mood or in the management of the diet. Try to make yourself understand the real motive for that desire for food. Is it true hunger, a physical need, a desire, or a response to an emotional state?

Try to put your attention on the "usefulness" of that food as a serving at that time compared to a serving postponed for a few days until the planned free meal when you can give in to whims.

Consciously decide whether to consume it or not at that time and if, for any reason, your choice will be to consume it, make it clear that it is a necessary act without guilt (better half a pack of cookies today than a pack a day for the next few days).

And if all this had not been served and impulse had prevailed over reason, it is necessary to acknowledge what happened by clearing away any sense of guilt and weakness ("I am not able," "I am weak," etc.), reasoning about the triggering factors, and considering the feelings experienced before and during the breakdown so as to learn how to exploit them in a positive way.

This will serve to understand how to improve and, above all, start immediately on the right foot beginning with the next meal. An occasional episode of diet-lapse will certainly not ruin everything that has been done on other days when you have commitment and dedication.

Finally, when planning a diet, do not forget to include moments to "train the mind" as well.

If you follow a restricted calorie diet, you know how difficult it is to be consistent with your food plan. Often, after having "sinned," we enter that tunnel of guilt and, from there, a vicious circle from which it is difficult to come out.

I know how difficult it is to be constant and to ignore all the temptations that call our attention, and especially our palate, every day.

I was there very often, too. So be quiet. Do not feel like a failure or one who fails to achieve his goals. We all have these periods. In those periods of high stress, it seems the only thing that can raise us is food. Sweet, salty, fried or breaded.

You know, when I started to change my lifestyle years ago, I often deliberately looked for situations where I could test my willpower. I went to birthday parties (but I ate first at home). I participated willingly in the parties in the classroom, where the only healthy thing was the salad of the super-stuffed sandwiches the caring mothers brought. I went out with those friends that I knew for sure would never have a healthy diet.

Do not get me wrong. There were more than a few nights that I had to deal with resisting Nutella crepes, fries, and other things.

Surely, you're thinking, "But, were you crazy?" Well, yes, maybe I was a little.

But in a sense, I enjoyed resisting all this. Despite that my dinner was low in carbohydrates and high in protein and that it was usually around 8 or 8:30 at night, I was determined to be constant. Every time I came home after that kind of evening, I felt proud of myself!

Unfortunately, as they say, it was not always all sunshine and rainbows. Sometimes, I wanted to say that it was "too much." I sometimes ended up really believing (yes, unfortunately, it happened) that I'd let myself be tempted by the first junk food I saw.

I told myself "just one, just to show that you are not fixed but that you only care about your health and your body." In the end, it went from one to two, then three, then four, to completely yielding to my temptation.

### *Those were the worst days.*

I felt like a failure, one who cannot resist his mind. Surely, you will understand me. Not because I want to give you the failure! I would never allow myself, but because we all face these obstacles sooner or later.

We all find ourselves in these situations! Here are a few tips that can help you to get a better mindset.

# 1. Tell your goals to someone.

When you have to be accountable to someone, things start to become much more serious.

Do you remember when, despite not wanting to, you did your homework? Then, you were accountable to someone (the teacher, your parents.) Even if doing homework was the most uncomfortable and tiresome thing in the world, you always ended with what was to be done.

It may seem absurd but accounting for something to someone allows you to have that consistency that otherwise you could hardly attain. When you need to do something just for yourself, take the matter very lightly, because there is no one who could scold you or judge you. But when you are subjected to judgments by others, you are assured that, before doing something that should not be done, you will think about it and think again, until you convince yourself that you really do not have to do it!

Whoever you want can be a good person to keep accountable to. Find someone who is really interested in you, like a parent, your boyfriend or girlfriend, and so on. The ideal would be to be accountable to a friend with whom you share this passion. We can better define it as your "Fit Buddy." Your Fit Buddy will be the person with whom you will undertake this path and with whom you will be constantly updating during your food day.

Establish a system of rewards and punishments with your fitness buddy, and each time one of you gives up, the other will have to give it a hard punishment. Be assured that this way, it will be easier to be constant and you will hardly be tempted to fall into temptation. Whatever it is.

## 2. Do not buy junk food when you shop.

Keeping temptations away is the first step to avoid falling into them.

The supermarket is one of the places where we are tempted the most. Passing next to shelves full of sweets and unhealthy foods put a strain on our determination. Well, here you will have to arm yourself with all your strength and focus only on the foods that are part of your diet. Do not linger there to look at brioches, cookies, etc., and think "I cannot eat them." Instead, think that by avoiding them, you will greatly improve your health.

If you are married and your husband does not follow diets and does not eat healthily, kindly ask him to hide all those foods that do not fit your diet, and that would distance you from achieving your goals. I believe that love is above all helping each other and what better situation than this to test his love for you.

If you really cannot ignore the temptations on the shelves of supermarkets or still prefer to stay away, you can do your shopping online. We asked the owner of an e-commerce company to do a whole category for us. The category is called "Gym Sickness," and in it, you can find all the fitness products you need to achieve your goal.

We know how difficult it is to resist the supermarket and to stand up against it, we have also thought about this.

## 3. Create healthy habits.

Good habits allow you to create the right conditions to progress in your goals and to be consistent in repeating them daily.

Replacing old and bad habits with new and healthy habits is not so simple. We have been used to unhealthy things for years and years. Our brain now performs them automatically, without wondering if it is right or wrong.

Some good habits could be:

- waking up early in the morning;
- going running;
- reading at least one book a month;
- drinking half a liter of water as soon as you wake up;

## 4. Read at least one motivational book a month.

Keeping your motivation alive is essential! I have read so many books in my adolescence. I was neither a nerd nor the first of the class, but I loved to read everything I thought interesting, and that deserved my attention.

Despite the many books on healthy eating, those that really helped me achieve my goals were those on motivation!

Reading all those success stories of people who have realized their dreams and goals gave me the charge to face up with all the difficulties that were on my way. All those beautiful motivational phrases helped me to plan the right mindset to become the person I wanted to be. I have read so many motivational and personal growth books. One thing is certain; this "category" will always remain my favorite.

## 6. Create a positive anchor whenever you resist temptation.

This is one of the techniques that fascinate me the most. The mind is something amazing and very powerful. Surely, you're wondering what these "positive anchors" are.

I want you to understand it for yourself. What is the anchor's job? To stay attached to the rock to allow the boat not to move, right? Okay, perfect. Imagine yourself as a great boat (not physically, of course). To remain stable, throw its anchors and grab a solid rock.

Whenever you say no to a temptation, whenever you can repel an invitation to dinner (knowing what will be waiting for you), whenever you go at the gym, whenever you have the strength to push yourself beyond your limits, whenever you are able to deal with a series of such things, you have to do something specific to remember to anchor that moment. It could be a gesture, eating food, a song, etc.

I'll give you an example: You're in front of the fridge, and you're opening it to get something you should not eat. Think back and close the fridge thinking that your goal is much more important than any delicacy. Good. At that moment, for example, hold your breath for a few seconds and watch your hand while doing it.

On such occasions, repeat this gesture several times. After a while, your mind will associate the gesture of the temptation to a moment of glory, and, every time you are about to break, you will just shake your hand to bring out the determination of that moment.

These are all anchors and are used in neuro-linguistic programming (NLP). Although it may seem absurd, I assure you that they are very powerful techniques used above all by the greatest champions.

For example, try to think of the gestures that the players do every time they score! Each of them has their own "move." That is their still positive. Using them will surely allow you to be consistent and focused.

## 7. Ask yourself why you do it and write the answer on a piece of paper.

Why are you doing it? I mean, why do you want to change your lifestyle? Why do you want to improve your body and your lifestyle?

If you do not have a real reason that pushes you to face all the various obstacles and sacrifices, you will leave at the first opportunity. But with this, I do not mean that if you do not have a super motivation, you will never reach your goals.

Motivation has to be really felt to be valid, and it can be anything you really want.

For example, you might be doing it for the following reasons:

- To be more beautiful;
- To please yourself more;
- As a child, they always took you around, but now, you want to show off who you are;
- You love to see tone and linear beautiful bodies so much that you would like yours to be the same.

Each of us has his own motivation! For example, mine was initially the desire to become an actor. I became interested in the world of fitness because I wanted to have a beautiful and perfect body just like that of the actors. From there, I discovered the linear and muscular bodies at the right point of fitness models and I fell in love with them. My focus has therefore shifted from wanting to have a dry body to wanting to have a tone and muscular body.

So, whatever your reason is, write it on a sheet of paper, hang it on the fridge, note it on your phone, do which one you want, but keep it in mind.

Trust me that you need to remember every day because doing all this will be a source of great motivation.

## 8. Have a diary and reflect each day on your journey.

One of the most effective tools to create a habit is a reflection. Having a diary in which to pen all our food intake is one of the best ways to reflect daily on what you really need to eat and what you did not need to eat. By doing so, you will be able to notice the obstacles that will arise along the way and decide how to overcome them. Knowing that you have to write in a diary what you eat in a day is a great incentive to promise to keep a list of healthy and fit meals and foods. Writing a food diary is certainly one of the best habits you can acquire.

Losing weight is not always easy. It is not because overweight and obesity are the results of several factors that intersect, overlap, and intertwine. Nutrition and physical conformation are the results of elements such as genetic, environmental, family, behavioral, and lifestyle. What matters, even more, is that behind these elements, there are mental, emotional, educational, and cultural causes that lead to behaving in one way or another.

In a research published in the Cochrane Review, it was found that diet is not sufficient to lose weight in the long term. It seems that less than 20% of obese people are able to lose 5% of their body weight and not recover it in the next 5 years.

It seems that the most effective weight loss program, in the long run, is one that combines diet, exercise, and psychological support. Furthermore, increasing the duration of psychological support further improves patient outcomes.

## Some Psychological Approaches to Weight Loss

Some psychological approaches have proved themselves useful for weight loss and maintenance of new body weight.

Cognitive behavioral therapy was created by Judith Beck based on the planning of what to eat, carefully organizing the purchase, the creation of the environment, the planning of "moments at risk", reminding the goals of weight loss every day, and the management of thoughts that impede weight loss.

Mindfulness-Based Mindfulness Therapy (MB-EAT) was designed by Jean Kristeller of Indiana University starting with the mindfulness-based stress reduction approach (MBSR) by Jon Kabat-Zinn and colleagues at Harvard University. It focuses on developing the innate wisdom about appetite and food. Mindfulness exercises teach people to turn their attention to the signs of the body, the hunger, the satiety, the taste, the consistency of what they want to eat. There is also an exposure phase in which people are faced with temptations. The focus is on satisfaction, the pleasure of eating more than on restriction. It seems this type of intervention is particularly effective in reducing emotional hunger and depression.

Biological and environmental factors. The factors that contribute to maintaining excess weight may differ from person to person. There is no magic recipe valid for everyone to lose weight. A study published in the Journal of Clinical Endocrinology and Metabolism found that leptin and ghrelin are able to identify obese people who are likely to reacquire weight after a diet. It is as if the brains of these people were more resistant to the stimuli of satiety. Other research has shown that people subject to emotional hunger, depression, or anxiety are more easily to regain weight. Correlations between childhood abuse and obesity have also been found. Environmental factors such as poverty, lack of access to healthy foods, sports, lack of time, and other cultural practices play a role in weight loss and physical fitness.

## Some Useful Strategies to Successfully Follow a Weight Loss Diet

Here, you can find some general tips that can be useful during your weight loss journey.

- Schedule an adequate amount of time each day to choose what to eat, buy it, cook it, and eat it.
- Keep a diary of the foods you eat, their amount, the changes in your body weight, the emotional and mental states related to meals
- Divide long-term goals into sub-goals to be verified in progress
- Draw lean ones after 6 or 12 months
- Have realistic expectations, one that is long-term, to be reassessed over time
- Think about all the activities that cannot be carried out because you're overweight and would like to practice once you have a leaner body.
- Do not perform activities simultaneously while eating
- Avoid heated discussions in the family or work at the restaurant
- Savor every single bite, trying to catch every little sensation
- Take care of the appearance of food like the presentation, colors, the table, lighting, and all that can enhance your appetite.
- Chew for a long time before swallowing.
- Take breaks from time to time and enjoy your favorite food

- Take time to just breathe and be with yourself.
- Pay attention to the mental and emotional states that are associated with food, choice, preparation, and consumption.
- Remove from the pantry, from drawers, etc. every unhealthy food
- Equip yourself with healthy snacks near you to avoid getting too hungry on the next meal.
- Always remember the goals of your weight loss and what drives us to do it.
- Do not dramatize in case of a snag, but consider it a possibility, but without becoming a systematic habit.
- Try to understand the reasons for the mischief and deal with it in another way that does not involve food.
- Celebrate your achievements in ways that do not contemplate food.
- Feed self-confidence, thank your motivation.
- Socialize with people who are experiencing a similar situation or who can still act as support and encouragement
- If necessary, ask a professional who can support you emotionally for help.
- Construct their time in creative, rewarding, and fulfilling activities
- Practice a sport you like, alone, or in a group

Eating is a necessary activity—the body is like a car, and without fuel, it cannot work. Unfortunately, in our society overloaded with food and obsessed with dieting, people build a relationship with extremely wrong foods, in which the act of eating becomes an automatic action and too often linked to negative emotions. In this chapter, I will try to explain to you the only thing you need to do to improve your relationship with food and make the act of eating an action that will not only bring nourishment but also pleasure.

Have you ever eaten food without even knowing what they are?

Do not worry. Unfortunately, it happens to many people. Every day, people come to my studio to tell me how they respond unconsciously to their food stimuli, always repeating the same actions and, above all, feeling deprived of the strength to change.

They tell me how often they do not derive any joy from what they eat and, on the contrary, gain a lot of frustration or guilt from it, and they want to know what they can do to improve their relationship with food. They have often tried everything and feel tired and disappointed.

The solution is actually much simpler than what you may believe.

The only thing you need to do to improve your relationship with food is not to do stressful diets (which only lower self-esteem) or spend whole days in the gym, but something much simpler. You have to become more aware of what you are doing.

Increasing awareness of your automated models can help you make more deliberate food choices and improve your relationship with food.

What you have to change is not so much the food you eat, but more on your relationship with it. Learning to eat with awareness will allow you to understand what your body really needs, and it will allow you to enjoy your meals.

In this way, you will reach your ideal weight without having to constantly resort to exasperating diets.

How do you do it?

Simple. You have to learn to be in contact with *you*!
You have to ask yourself some good questions to help you become aware of the hundreds of food decisions you take every day without even realizing it.

Here are some good questions you must ask yourself to become more aware and improve your relationship with food.

1. Why do I eat?

This is the main question that will guide all your future decisions. And in the vast majority of cases, you do not know why you're eating! People hardly stop to wonder what drives them to go to the kitchen and open the pantry drawer. Many times, one believes that they are hungry, but in reality, they only feel like that in response to an emotional stimulus, such as boredom or stress. Learning to recognize this difference is the first step to effectively fight your urges and discover the real needs of your body. Take a break to ask yourself, "Am I really hungry?" Whenever you feel like you need to eat, it will help you differentiate your physical hunger from environmental and emotional stimuli.

2. When do I eat?

If you have ever followed a diet in your life, you will have realized that the traditional dietary approaches do nothing but provide you with a food plan where they tell you what you should eat, how much you have to eat, and what time you have to eat! This cannot be more wrong. These rules do nothing but disconnect you from your natural nourishment needs and only encourage you to ignore internal signals of hunger and satiety.

3. What do I eat?

Diets are definitely frustrating. They force you to eliminate a lot of things, and often, the best ones in terms of taste! To be able to do this, you are required to have a certain willpower that must be maintained for a very long time, which is very difficult even for the most persevering people. Learning to consume a little of everything in a moderate way, ranging from healthier foods to those that you eat for pleasure, will lead you to live your relationship with food in a much more balanced way. By freeing yourself from restrictions, you will develop the ability to respond to the wisdom of your body—that innate wisdom that is within each person.

4. How do I eat?

Quickly? Standing up? Watching TV? Many people eat this way and are so inclined to eat more—this feeling of satiety and satisfaction is, in fact, less when not paying attention to the food you introduce. Learn to avoid multitasking when you eat and dedicate quality time to the activity of eating. In this way, you will be able to feel what your body has to tell you, such as when it is time to stop, so as to avoid the binge you will later regret.

5. How much do you eat?

Normally, classic diets focus on how much you are allowed to eat using methods based on the control of calories or fat.

This behavior, however, in the long run, leads you to spend an enormous amount of time, energy, and willpower. Turning the meal into a mechanical experience will make you disconnect from internal signals, and this will favor problematic behaviors rather than reducing them. Paying attention to the signs of satiety and determining small goals in the situation such as feeling better after eating than before you start will make you able to eat the "right" amount of food based on the real needs of your body. For example, young children eat when they are hungry and stop when they are full. They touch, smell, and explore food while eating it. Re-learning these innate behaviors in humans is essential for developing a healthy relationship with food.

The idea of starting a diet can be daunting, especially if you are not mentally prepared to face such a change. When the mind is calm and prepared, sticking to a healthy food program is much simpler. With the right preparation, you will be able to effectively achieve your goals, and you will make it less difficult not to fall into temptation during the journey.

Be aware of the recurring negative thoughts related to food.

Oftentimes, our diets fail because of our beliefs related to food and eating. Try to become aware of your food beliefs and make an effort to change your mentality.

We often think that on special occasions, it is right to let go a bit. There's nothing wrong with eating a little more from time to time, but be honest with yourself about what you consider "special occasions." When events like eating away from home, business lunches, office parties, and other small events all become excuses to let yourself binge, the failure of the diet is just around the corner. Therefore, try to re-evaluate what occasions can be considered as "special" and when it is better to stick to your original diet plan.

Do you use food as a reward?

Many think that after a long busy day, it is normal to deserve to go out for dinner or eat an entire tub of ice cream. Look for alternative ways to reward yourself which do not include food. For example, take a long hot bath, buy a new dress, or go to the cinema. There are many ways to reward yourself without using food.

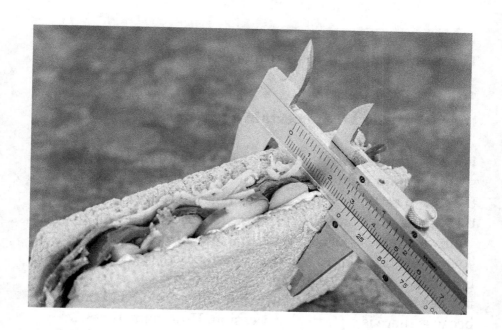

# The Importance of Listening to your Body

## Dissociate food from certain activities.

Food is closely linked to numerous social rituals. Giving up sugar and fat may not be easy when we emotionally associate them with certain habits. Make a conscious effort to break these dangerous patterns, as they can become a big obstacle to your weight loss journey. With this, there is a tendency to consume larger quantities of unhealthy food, especially during holidays. For instance, it is pretty common for people to indulge in cakes and pastries, even if they are on diet, just because there is a particular occasion. How many times we have heard people saying that they will start their diet on January first? Hundreds, if not thousands. The reality is that there is no need to wait until a specific day to start a die. The sooner you will start learning new and healthier habits, the sooner you will begin to see results.

With this, we are not saying you should not enjoy a piece of cake on your birthday or during special occasions. We are just pointing out the fact that associating "fun" and "happiness" with processed foods can be detrimental for your weight loss. Being "aware" of this trap is the first step to become healthier and, more importantly, to know when it is time to "let go" and indulge in what you like the most and when it is better to take a step back and realize what you are trying to do.

Try to be aware of the times you eat too much or make bad food choices, both in terms of food and the things you drink. Whenever you go to the cinema, do you buy Coca-Cola and popcorn? Cannot say "no" to a few glasses of wine during the evenings out? Cannot imagine a Saturday morning without coffee and donuts? If so, take the extra mile to commit to cutting these associations.

Try changing associations by replacing harmful foods with healthier ones. For example, when you spend the evening out, dedicate it to a board game instead of focusing on drinking. On Saturday mornings, have breakfast with coffee, yogurt, and fresh fruits. If, at the end of the day you tend to try to relax through eating, replace the food with a good book or some music.

## It is not just about calories.

In the end, you will be more likely to be able to stick to your diet by committing yourself to change your negative behaviors rather than just keeping your calories under control. Try to become aware of when you eat and why you do it. Even if it is only half a biscuit, ask yourself if you are allowing it because you think you have had a bad day. Do you tend to eat because you are hungry or because you feel bored? If you do it out of boredom, try to get rid of this bad habit. Even if you do not exceed the calories you can consume in a day, always try to use common sense. Do not eat the wrong foods for the wrong reasons, because it is the fastest way to associate pleasure with food, which is something you have to avoid at all costs if you want to lose weight successfully.

**Ask for help.**

Changing is not easy, and sometimes, we are not able to do it on our own. Ask for help from friends and family. Let them know you are trying to lose weight and pray to support yourself. Make sure they know they do not have to invite you to parties where cheap food and alcohol will be served. Share your goals with all the people living under your own roof.

**Establish contained and realistic goals.**

Many people tend to sabotage their diet by placing the bar of expectations too high. Set achievable goals if you want to be able to stick to your plans.

Remember that a balanced diet allows you to lose about ½-1 kilo a week, no more. If you intend to lose weight faster than that, prepare to fail.

Initially, you should have cautious goals, so you will be more likely to be able to reach them and have the motivation to continue. Unspecific intentions such as "This week, I will eat vegetables every day," and something like, "The next time I eat out of the house, I will order a salad instead of potato chips," are valid starting points that can lead you to the road to success.

**Keep a diary of what you eat.**

If you want your diet to be successful, you cannot exempt yourself from being responsible. Go out and buy a diary that will accompany you along the entire route. Record everything you eat every day and keep a calorie count. A tangible account will force you to notice your bad habits and motivate you to develop new ones.

## Plan your meals.

Planning meals and snacks in advance will help you not to give in to temptations. In the days before the start of the diet, make a list of healthy recipes that you intend to prepare. Try to get ahead, for example, by buying or cutting the necessary ingredients. If you want, you can also cook soups and vegetables to keep in the refrigerator—they will be very useful for the first week lunches.

## Focus on concrete behavior.

When you limit yourself to making analyses in abstract terms, it will not be easy to develop greater willpower. Examining your concrete actions will help you start the transformation. Make a list of the wrong habits you want to change. Start with small, gradual changes. Try to commit yourself to abandon an old behavior for a week, and then continue making new changes slowly.

For example, you decide that after work, you will walk for 40 minutes rather than watching a show. Commit to respecting your purpose for a week. In the following days, you can gradually increase the duration of the exercise, e.g. by walking for an hour.

On the occasions when the willpower is not yet sufficient, commit to bringing yourself back to the right path, even if it may mean having to be particularly hard on yourself. Doing so will help you understand that you are the only one who has the power to change your behavior.

Recognize and admit your failures. Register them on your food diary. Take responsibility for your failure, learn from it, and grow stronger.

Describe the reasons that led to failure, highlighting your disappointment. For example, write something like, "At dinner, I ate dessert because I chose to, and I felt guilty after doing it." Although they may sound harsh words, many believe that saying them is useful to express clearly that they have failed. You will feel motivated to make greater efforts to be able to change.

For some, taking a weekly meal "out of the rules" can be a valid help to stay on track. A deprivation that has lasted too long may cause the whole project to go up in smoke. Sticking to a strict diet may seem more feasible when you know that at the end of the tunnel, you can give yourself the coveted food. If you think it might be useful to check you, consider scheduling a premium meal at the end of the week.

## Three Meals a Day Is Not the Best Solution

Why do we eat what we eat? The simpler answer is that we choose to eat what we like. And it is a correct answer: satisfaction is the main factor influencing our food choices. But the question is more complex. Scientific literature has highlighted a link between food and the expression of both social and personal identity—we are what we eat, not only in biological terms but also in symbolic terms. In fact, food practices refer to the different collective belonging and manifest the individual adherence to a lifestyle. Moreover, social psychology, in explaining human behavior, takes into account the fact that we do not live in isolation but together with other people who inevitably influence us. Therefore, in addition to the tastes and information we possess (for example, on the presumed healthiness of certain foods), the influence of others also contributes to determining our eating habits, often through the identification processes with different social groups. Without claiming to be exhaustive, let's look at some examples of social influence on eating behavior.

The first to influence us are certainly our parents, especially our mothers, who can condition us in different ways. First of all, through their example, our mothers are the first models we imitate in general and also with regard to the relationship with food. When we were in their womb, we began to taste and learn about the flavors of our family and our culture. This selective exposure to food continues throughout the period of breastfeeding (even our mothers' milk takes the taste of what they eat) and continues for a long time. In fact, at least until the children reach 11-12 years old, our parents decide which foods come into the pantry and arrive at the table. This type of influence is fundamental because the selection of the food we are experiencing greatly influences our tastes, which are mainly formed through simple exposure and repeated experience. They are built on familiarity—we like what we are used to eating.

A second way by which tastes develop is through associations that are established between certain food and a positive or negative situation. Parents can also influence these associations. If the family meal is a nice moment and an opportunity for sharing and living peacefully, our relationship with food will be connoted in a positive sense. If the meal is a battlefield, a place of conflict in which they force us to eat something that does not go well, then our relationship with food will perhaps be compromised and will haunt us even into adulthood.

Growing up, our peers become increasingly important both in general and as sources of influence on our eating behavior. Our peers influence us because we tend to imitate them. For example, at the end of a dinner with new friends, we often ask ourselves, "Should I get the dessert?" It may happen that we have a great desire for it, but if nobody takes it, we will probably give it up. Some research shows that people eat less if they are together with people who eat little and eat more if they are together with people who eat a lot. Why does this happen? In general, there are two fundamental reasons. On the one hand, if we do not know how to behave in a certain situation, which is perhaps new and unusual, we look at what others do to understand what is the appropriate behavior, and we repeat it. We also imitate others because we identify with them and we want to feel accepted or at least not seem strange or deviant. This is where the idea of having 3 meals a day came from. As we will see in the next chapters, however, it is not the best solution.

As you can see, the importance of the mindset is very high and it is safe to say that without the proper mindset, it is impossible to be successful with the ketogenic diet. This, however, opens the doors for something interesting. In fact, if we have the power within our own mind to be successful, it means that the outside world does not have an impact on our ability to be skinnier in the future. Most people that are currently overweight or that are trying to get back in shape, often times, blame their circumstances or even other people to make up for their failure. However, now that we have understood the important role played by our mind during a weight loss phase, it is safe to say that we can take on full responsibility for our weight and we can become the real master of our bodies. When you realize that you are in full control of what you eat and how many calories you consume in a day, you can decide what you are going to do about your situation. If you listen closely to the stories of the successful people that have lost an incredible number of pounds or kilos, you will see that each and every one of them started by realizing they were the only people to hold responsible for their situation. Yes, genetics and other factors can play a role, but if you truly want to achieve a result, you will be able to get the body of your dreams. This is an invitation to grow stronger and become a new person through weight loss and, to be more specific, through the adoption of a ketogenic lifestyle. If you decide to make a positive change, you can be sure that the people around you, those who really care about your health, will be more than happy to support along your journey in becoming a better and fitter version of yourself.

# Chapter 2: Basics of the Ketogenic Diet

Before getting into the details of the ketogenic diet, we would like to spend some time talking about the basics of nutrition. It is fundamental to understand the basic concepts, before diving deeper into the topic. When we talk about diet and nutrition, we often do not know the principles that underlie our very existence and, above all, our physical well-being. We limit ourselves to eating something that others have advised us, and we often take advertised pills and tablets which not only have no use but can even be harmful to our health and our finances.

In order not to get lost in the complicated world of nutrition, the first useful thing to do is an overview of food principles and daily human needs. This chapter will give you all the information you need to have a complete understanding of how your body works and how food can have a relevant impact on its efficiency.

Let's start by saying that all foods can be classified into five large food groups:

- carbohydrates
- proteins (or protides)
- fats (or lipids)
- vitamins
- minerals

Carbohydrates are the nutrients most present in our diet. They are made up of two main elements—carbon and water—that when joined together give rise to the simplest of sugars, glucose. Aggregating them into larger molecules, they form two different groups of carbohydrates: simple sugars (consisting of a few molecules of glucose) and complex sugars (formed by long chains of glucose). A subsequent classification is that which divides them into monosaccharides (a sugar molecule), disaccharides (two molecules), and polysaccharides (more than two molecules). To be honest, things get much more complicated, but there is no need to be too scientific, especially if you just want to lose weight.

There are about 200 different types of carbohydrates, and often times, they take the name from the food in which they are in large quantities. For instance, there are some carbohydrates called fructose, lactose, maltose, but also sucrose and starch. Carbohydrates can be found mainly in vegetables, and their function is purely energetic and makes up the basis of human nutrition—providing about 4 calories per gram/weight. They are found in large quantities in pasta, rice, potatoes, fruit, milk, bread, flour, as well as in legumes.

They are the most famous nutrient since they are contained in so many foods.

The cells of our body transform all the carbohydrates introduced into the simplest form, glycogen, which, once oxidized into the cellular mitochondria, provides energy for rapid and clean use, i.e. without waste. These must, therefore, represent the basis of our nutrition and must provide about 60-65% of the energy needs.

However, it is rare to have to carry out a glucosidic supplementation. In fact, they are so widely present in all foods that perhaps we should think about reducing their consumption.

Fats, on the other hand, are complex acidic structures found in both animal and vegetable foods. Like carbohydrates, fats also have a purely energetic function with different caloric value. Lipids bring about 9 calories per gram/weight, and their burning rate is very slow. In fact, before being used, fats must be transformed into simpler elements, which the cell can then oxidize to obtain energy. In their complex form, on the other hand, they are easily stored as fat storage, which is the energy reserve of our body. Fats are often divided into saturated and unsaturated, depending on the type of chemical bond that forms the molecule. To simplify, we can say that saturated fats are "bad" and harmful to our arteries—these include cholesterol, glycerol, hydrogenated fats, fats contained in butter and margarine, palm oil, and most fats of animal origin.

The "good" fats instead are the unsaturated fats or those contained in olive oils and in many seed oils, fish fats (omega 3 and omega 6), and lecithin (abundant in soybeans).

In addition to energy capacity, fats are involved in many organic activities including hormone synthesis and cell membrane construction. Therefore, their function is vital, and our energy needs should be covered by lipids in the measure of 15-20%. This means that only 20% of the daily calories consumed should be fats, possibly good ones.

The integration of fats is very rare, as we usually tend to consume more than we should since they are the vehicle of taste and make us better appreciate the foods we ingest.

When it comes to proteins, it is a totally different story. They are composed of complex chains of amino acids joined together by peptide bonds. These amino acids can bind together in number, proportions, and different forms—giving rise to an almost infinite series of specific proteins.

There are 21 amino acids, 8 of which are called "essential," because our body is not able to synthesize them. In fact, human RNA possesses protein synthesis codes for only 13 amino acids and is able to process proteins that contain only these elements. For a complete protein range, it is necessary to take the remaining 8 amino acids, called essential, from the outside through eating.

Animal and vegetable proteins are made of the same amino acids—with a substantial difference. While each animal protein contains all 21 amino acids (in different proportions, depending on the protein itself), in the proteins coming from vegetables, there is always something missing. Some plant foods, therefore, contain certain amino acids but do not contain others. It becomes important, then, in the case of a vegetarian diet, to know how to combine the various products so that all the necessary elements are introduced. As we said, this does not apply to animal proteins, which are called "noble" because they are complete.

From an energetic point of view, protides are similar to carbohydrates, bringing about 4 calories per gram/weight. Unfortunately, the energy obtained from proteins is not as clean, because nitrogen is released as a result of oxidation at the cellular level, which then evolves into free radical, accelerating the cellular aging process.

The energetic process of proteins is just a fallback of the body in the event of an actual need for calories. Normally, protides are used for "plastic" purposes, i.e. they are used in the construction, repair, and renewal of all body structures such as muscles, bones, cells, organs, apparatuses, and tissues. It can be said that the human body is composed of 70% water and the rest of it is proteins. To maintain itself, the human body, therefore, needs a certain daily protein intake, which should be about one gram per kilogram of body weight (a man of 80 kilograms should take 80 grams of protein per day). However, this proportion can range between 0.70 grams per kilogram/weight (the minimum to remain healthy) up to a maximum of 1.5 grams per kilogram/weight. Beyond this threshold, there is the risk that the proteins you eat cause the development of many free radicals and other problems related to kidneys and liver. Ultimately, the daily caloric intake of proteins should be 15-20%.

The supplementation of proteins may be necessary in the case of a vegetarian diet (for the speech of amino acids), while it is almost never recommended in the case of a varied diet that also includes foods of animal origin. Moreover, the assimilation of protides for plastic use is about 4 grams per hour, so we can assume that the body has more means of using them for energy. However, the proteins taken through supplements are less similar than those taken through normal nutrition, as they are metabolized with a certain amount of carbohydrates and vitamins (especially B12).

Another important part of nutrition is the macro group of vitamins. They are organic compounds essential to life and development that normally the human body cannot synthesize, and therefore, must take with food. They are found in large quantities in vegetables, fruit, milk, and its derivatives. Many vitamins are sensitive to high temperatures, so it is advisable to take these foods raw. Moreover, some of them deteriorate over time and becoming bioavailable. This is why it is preferable to eat freshly picked fruits and vegetables.

Each vitamin has a specific function, which can vary from the metabolic one (e.g. B12) to the one protecting the blood vessels (vitamin C). The deficiency of a certain vitamin, usually called avitaminosis, can cause specific diseases such as scurvy in the case of vitamin C deficiency. This is why it is important to have a balanced diet in terms of vitamins intake.

Vitamins are distinguished between two categories namely water-soluble (which mean they can be melted in water) and liposoluble (melted in fats).
Our body is able to store the fat-soluble vitamins (A, D, E, K, and F), while it cannot retain the water-soluble vitamins (C, B1, B2, B5, B6, B12, H, PP) that are easily eliminated in the urine.
The latter, in fact, should be taken several times throughout the day. It is also worthy to note that fat-soluble vitamins, which are stored in body fat, have a slower process of elimination. This can cause, in the case of high intake, a state of toxicity, thus creating very serious dysfunctions. Therefore, if the integration of water-soluble vitamins can be made lightly, we must instead pay maximum attention when it comes to the fat-soluble ones, which should be integrated only in case of established deficiency.

The last food group is one of the minerals and inorganic elements (i.e. without biological carbon) that cover multiple functions. They are often called mineral salts, but this is an improper name since most minerals are devoid of the salt part. Rather, they are single elements present in nature—metals and non-metals—which use water as a vehicle to pass from the earth to the plants, and therefore, to the animals that feed on them.

They are divided into three groups called macro-elements, micro-elements, and oligo-elements. This division is established on the basis of the daily requirement of the elements, which can vary from 100 milligrams/day for the macro-elements (calcium, phosphorus, potassium, etc.), to less than 200 micrograms/day for the oligo-elements (manganese, chromium, cobalt, etc.)

Although their presence in the body is around 5%/6% of the body weight, they are of vital importance, as they participate in many cellular and metabolic functions.
For instance, just think about iron which plays an important part in the cardiovascular system or calcium which is a fundamental element of bones and teeth. They must be eaten on a regular basis, as the body expels them through urine, feces, and sweat.

A varied diet, in which vegetables, fruit, milk, meat, fish, eggs, and dried fruit are added, provides the optimal amount of all the necessary minerals.

Mineral deficiency, just like vitamins, can lead to specific diseases such as iron deficiency, anemia, or it can even aggravate diseases such as osteoporosis in the case of calcium deficiency. Therefore, a certain quantity of minerals is vital. But excess quantities can lead to of poisoning. Hence, it would be good to stay away from the saline and mineral supplements, unless there's an ascertained shortage. Most importantly, before starting the intake through supplements, it is advisable to seek medical advice.

After reading these pages, you now have a complete understanding of how nutrition works and how you can use the different elements to create a sustainable meal plan. In the ketogenic diet, all the calories will be assumed mainly from proteins and fats over a short period of time, but it is still crucial to have a balanced ratio of the different nutrients. At first, it all may seem complicated, but once you go through the rest of the book, you will have a much clearer picture of what to do to be successful with the ketogenic diet.

In the following pages, we are going to discuss what the ketogenic diet is and why it is becoming more and more popular these days. In fact, just by browsing the web for a few minutes, it is easy to find articles and blogs dedicated to this topic. Most people, however, decide to follow the diet without knowing what they are getting themselves into and are not able to distinguish good information from that which is harmful. This is why we decided to start the book by laying out the foundation of this diet, allowing everybody to understand its principles. Let's get started!

If there is a diet whose nature and modality are often misunderstood, it is the ketogenic diet. Exalted by some as a very effective means of weight loss, demonized by others for the supposed – and often exaggerated – risks that are ascribed to it, it is actually an important tool in a whole series of situations. It is a particular diet that must be used with due precautions and diligence, but which can guarantee relevant results where other methods often fail.

The premise upon which the ketogenic diet is based is the ability of our body to use lipid reserves with great effectiveness when the availability of carbohydrates is greatly reduced. The physiological mechanisms activated in this situation reduce the possible use of proteins for energy, protecting the lean mass and significantly reducing the sensation of hunger.

In the clinical field, the first documented use of a ketogenic diet to treat specific diseases dates back to the 1920s when Doctor Wilder used it to control attacks in pediatric patients with epilepsy that was not treatable with the then available drugs. Its use returned to the again in the 1990s, and since then, it spread more and more. In the 60s and 70s, with the constant increase of overweight and obese subjects, numerous studies were carried out on the use of a low-calorie diet that could lead to a rapid and significant weight reduction without affecting the lean mass.

The various protocols of PSMF (Protein Sparing Modified Fast) were born, diets characterized by a reduced protein intake with the almost total absence of carbohydrates and a measured protein intake aimed at minimizing the loss of precious muscle mass. The spread of the ketogenic diet saw a surge with the appearance on the market of low-carb diets and do-it-yourself diets. One clear example of this is the Atkins diet, a model that drastically reduces the consumption of carbohydrates, allowing instead, to eat fat freely and proteins.

It is a grotesque caricature of the ketogenic diet based on improbable and fanciful interpretations of human physiology, rightly criticized by the entire scientific community.

In recent times, the emergence of the Paleo Diet has brought back into the diet food regimens the reduced carbohydrate content that can generate ketosis. Here, solid scientific basis intertwines with perturbed, poorly-engineered biological concepts that have often generated grotesque solutions in which every carbohydrate is demonized and considered a poison, while the consumption of bacon is recommended, food which was notoriously abounded in the Paleolithic era.

In recent years, there has been a renewed interest by the scientific community toward the Paleo Diet, with the use of ketogenic choices for the treatment of obesity and for other diseases such as certain forms of tumors, some neurological diseases like Alzheimer's and Parkinson's, Diabetes, and the Metabolic Syndrome. The human organism has several forms of accumulation of reserves of which the most consistent is represented by the adipose tissue. In an average individual weighing 70 kg, the total adipose tissue can amount to about 15 kg, while the carbohydrate portion amounts to less than half of a kilogram.

It is evident that the sugar reserves can guarantee energy for very limited periods of time, while fats represent a huge reserve of energy. Tissues receive energy in proportion to the actual availability of substrates in the blood. When glucose is present in sufficient quantities, then it appears to be the preferred energy source for most of the body tissues. When glucose is in short supply, most organs and tissues can use fatty acids as an energy source or can convert other substances into sugars, especially some amino acids such as alanine and glutamine through a process called gluconeogenesis.

Some organs and tissues, such as the brain, the Central Nervous System, red blood cells, and type II muscle fibers, are not able to use free fatty acids, but under the conditions of glucose deficiency, can use ketone bodies. These are substances derived from lipidic parts, the concentration of which is usually very small under normal conditions but raises considerably in particular situations such as a prolonged fasting or a long period without carbohydrate introduction.

The increase in the concentration of ketone bodies in the blood resulting from fasting or severe reduction of their intake with the diet is a completely natural condition called ketosis, a mechanism evolved to cope with the stringent metabolic needs and limited availability of food of our hunter-gatherer's past, naturally also present in the morning after the nocturnal fasting or after intense and prolonged physical and muscular efforts.

The severe restriction of carbohydrate intake, through action on hormones such as insulin and glucagon, promotes the mobilization of lipids from the reserve tissues and their use for energy purposes. Given the scarcity of glucose, the present acetyl-CoA is used for the production of ketone bodies, substances such as acetone, acetoacetate, and Î2-hydroxybutyric acid, which become the preferred fuel for the cells of the Central Nervous System. During ketosis, blood sugar is maintained at normal levels thanks to the use of glucogenic amino acids and glycerol derived from the demolition of triglycerides to form glucose.

In physiological ketosis, the presence of ketone bodies in the blood passes from 0.1 mmol/dl to about 7 mmol/dl, without, determining significant alteration of the pH which normally stays around 7.4. However, it may decrease slightly in the first days, given the acidity of ketone bodies, to return quickly to normal levels as long as the concentration of ketone bodies remains less than 10 mmol/dl.

The effect of saving protein reserves could occur through different mechanisms. The use of proteins is important in the first days of the diet, but as the body begins to predominantly use free fatty acids and ketones for their energy needs, the demand for glucose drops drastically accompanied by the reduction of the use of amino acids for energy purposes. A direct effect of the ketone bodies on the protein metabolism and on the action of the thyroid is not excluded, with a reduction of T3.

The excess ketones that are not used at the level of the tissues are eliminated through breathing in the form of acetone, which results in bad breath, and through the urine, where excess acidity is buffered by simultaneous elimination of sodium, potassium, and magnesium.

Ketosis determines changes in the concentration of different hormones and nutrients, including ghrelin, amylin and leptin and, of course, ketone bodies. It is probably through these variations that one of the most relevant effects of the ketogenic diet is determined. The reduction or total disappearance of the sensation of hunger that is typical in ketosis, undoubtedly, a situation that better help to endure the typical rigor of this diet.

## The Science behind the Ketogenic Diet

Do you like to follow a diet that would allow you to lose fat at maximum speed, and in the same span of time, allow you to maintain and gain new muscle mass? Well, I and some of my friends found a diet that does just that. We just followed a cyclic ketogenic diet. This is virtually a sado-maso diet, dedicated to those who embrace certain sufferings. But I can guarantee you that it works great.

To me, and to all those who followed this diet, it gave amazing results. It was one of the two diets experimented with the Ultimate America competition, and it really gave exceptional results even to those without a champion metabolism. But it requires grit. The basic principle is simple. The body uses the main source of energy available as fuel. Under normal conditions, the preferred fuel of the body comes from carbohydrates.

When you are on a diet, once the carbohydrates are gone, the body will convert part of the muscle protein into glucose (because the body requires it) which can result to the loss of muscle mass. If instead, you follow a rich protein diet, these will be largely converted into glucose by a process called glucogenesis and, once again, when the food proteins are consumed, the body will convert part of the muscle protein into glucose (because the body requires glucose, even in the face of inevitable loss of muscle mass).

However, if there was a way to change the body's fuel, then the muscle proteins would be preserved. The ketogenic diet dramatically succeeds in this purpose. Fats become the main source of energy and, once the fat is consumed (since the body no longer requires energy as glucose but fat in the form of ketones), ketones will be converted into energy for the body.

After about 20 years of absence, the ketogenic diet has reappeared both in the slimming sector and in sports nutrition. In America (home from which food discoveries are born, both valid and useless), books like *Dr. Atkins New Diet Revolution*, *Protein Power* by Eades, and, albeit with less emphasis, *The Carbohydrate Addicts Diet* by Hellers, have brought back a low carbohydrate diet. Furthermore, in the sector of sports nutrition, two more but slightly different methods have come to public attention.

We are talking about *The Anabolic Diet* by Dr. Mauro Di Pasquale and *Bodyopus* created by Dan Duchaine. These two systems do not propose following a carbohydrate-free diet to the bitter end. Rather, they are based on a system that provides five days almost without carbohydrates alternating with two days of carbohydrate refill, a model used by athletes before a race.

Mauro di Pasquale and Dan Duchaine have written two small books about it that I would define as "incomplete ideas." I have read them at least 10 times each and from those bases, I started experimenting. Now, without false modesty, I can say that I think I am one of the absolute people who know the most. I have been on the ketogenic diet, alternately, for about three years. I studied books, articles, and anything I found on the web. Then I experimented with them. I performed ketogenic in all sauces and in all ways. For around six months, I measured my blood sugar five times a day until I got to the point of knowing automatically how much my glycemia increased with a meal and how much it would be lowered in how much time. In the next chapters, I will talk about how to put it into practice. I will talk about the target ketogenic diet and all the tricks to be applied to the ketogenic diet.

## What are ketones?

The term ketosis, or acidosis, indicates a biological process linked to metabolism and nutrition.

In very simple terms, when the body goes down on glucose or on blood sugar, it tends to compensate for this lack of energy with increased production of free ketone bodies at the blood level. What are ketone bodies and what does their concentration mean?

These are molecules of a lipid nature synthesized by the liver, but they have metabolic characteristics similar to those of sugars. This is why, under particular conditions, the brain stimulates greater production of free ketones. This concentration of ketogenic bodies produces acetone which can be evident in having a bad. In fact, the brain's reaction is simply an emergency strategy.

## When are we at risk of going into ketosis?

The causes can be different. Some are pathological, while others are induced by the diet. Among those linked to morbid conditions we surely find diabetes, pancreas or liver diseases, or alcoholism. However, recently, there is often talk of ketogenic diets, which cause acidosis in the body in a deliberate way, even if not for prolonged periods (because the health would be compromised otherwise). These are unbalanced and high-protein diet, in which, the intake of carbohydrates (simple and complex) and sugars is totally absent. This should induce weight loss, and it is no coincidence that ketosis also occurs during periods of fasting.

In my opinion, this is a good solution even if the diet is short-lived. Ketogenic bodies pass into the urine and through the kidneys. It is true that they may lead to dehydration, muscle fatigue, and cramps, but studies have shown that it is sufficient to drink a lot of water during the day to stay healthy. To restore normal metabolic conditions and regain strength, we must, therefore, reintroduce mineral salts and glucose into the diet, or administer insulin if ketosis is induced by diabetes or pancreatic diseases.

**The ketogenic index:** Food can be classified as ketogenic or antiketogenic depending on their ability to convert to glucose in the blood. Foods that are primarily made of fats are the most ketogenic element because they can only be converted to 10% glucose. Proteins are in the middle because they can be converted into glucose with a capacity of 58%. Carbohydrates are converted into glucose with 100% efficacy and are naturally antiatherogenic.

The ketogenic index indicates how much a diet promotes ketosis and can be calculated with the following formula:

$$KR = (0.9 * F + 0.46 * P) / (1.0 * C + 0.1 * F + 0.58 * P)$$

F = indicates the total grams of fat supplied by the diet
P = indicates the total grams of proteins supplied by the diet
C = indicates the total grams of carbohydrates provided by the diet

A ketogenic index equal to or greater than 1.5 promotes a rapid establishment of the state of ketosis.

## What exactly does it mean to be in a ketosis state?

Ketosis simply indicates a metabolic state in which the concentration of ketone bodies in the blood is greater than the concentration of glucose. However, this is not to be compared to the ketoacid state that occurs in diabetic subjects.

Being in ketosis involves two things:

1. The power of the metabolism of fats has been activated.
2. The entire fat degradation system is in perfect condition and is efficient.

Usually, the state of ketosis is a source of concern for doctors. However, unless you are in serious medical conditions like diabetes; excess ketones are easily pushed out the body through the urine. This permits a person to control the intensity of ketosis which can e monitored using Ketosticks.

The ideal time to measure your ketosis level is in the morning, as during the day, the ketones could be used entirely for energy purposes, and therefore, may not be detected by the Ketostick.

## Effects on the Metabolism of the Ketogenic Diet

The creation of a ketosis state, even for small periods of time, increases the body's ability to use fat as fuel. Furthermore, glucose oxidation decreases as the ketone bodies provide most of the energy the organism needs. In addition, a ketogenic diet improves the ability to oxidize fats even in well-trained athletes.

One argument for discussion is whether the ketogenic diet favors or not saving the body proteins compared to a diet of equal calories but high in carbohydrates. Several studies seem to try saving protein. Other reliable data from observations seem to support the idea that the ketogenic diet prevents proteins from being used as an energy source.

Since there is an almost unlimited source of fats in the body that can convert into ketones, and since they can be oxidized by every tissue, there is no request for the body to convert proteins into glucose by glucogenesis. However, it is appropriate for a normal person to take at least 1 gram of protein x kilogram of body weight. While for an athlete, 2.2 grams x kg of body weight is ideal. It is good not to exceed 2.5 grams because, as already mentioned, some amino acids are converted into glucose, causing an insulin reaction.

## Other Effects of Low Carbohydrates Diets

It has been proven that an almost carbohydrate-free diet will allow greater lipolysis and a greater release of glycerol compared to a normal or high carbohydrate diet. This is due to the total lack of insulin, which blocks lipolysis even at small concentrations and the fact that the production of GH (growth hormone) is increased, which also has a lipolytic action and also increases glucagon, catecholamines, and glucocorticoids.

The increase in the amount of growth hormone, due to the ketogenic diet, not only promotes lipolysis but also prevents the inevitable loss of protein that would instead occur with a normal low-calorie diet.

I hope you now understand what happens when a condition of ketosis is established through the abolition of carbohydrates and an appropriate ratio between fats and proteins, and training. All this suggests that the reduction of insulin, combined with the new hormonal condition, maximize the oxidation of fats. However, some lucky individuals are able to obtain excellent results without reaching such extreme diets. It is also possible to improve the hormonal pattern through some small tricks.

For example, decreasing the number of carbohydrates consumed and making use of foods with a low glycemic index in place of carbohydrates with a high glycemic index will lower the level of insulin. It can also help to ingest foods rich in fiber. You can also never eat carbohydrates alone but combine them with fats and proteins (such as the 40/30/30 diet). This favors a more gradual release of blood glucose and a balance between insulin and glucagon.

So far, we have discussed what the ketogenic diet is. But what interests the athletes is not so much a continuous keto regimen, but more of a cyclic keto regimen. What is this? It is a diet that consists of a period of total deprivation of

---

carbohydrates with only a few days where you do a refill of carbohydrates. In fact, the issue with every diet is the consequential loss of muscle tissue.

Loss of muscles is also a cause of slowed metabolism. Although the ketogenic diet is the most effective way to prevent the loss of contractile proteins (muscles), it is possible that some muscle tissue is lost just the same if you continue this type of diet indefinitely. This is why two days high in calories and rich in carbohydrates fill the reservoirs of glycogen muscles (for training in the next week) again and stimulate anabolism and promote muscle growth.

What science still cannot explain is why the two days of high carbohydrates do not modify the metabolic adaptations stimulated by ketosis. It would seem possible because it takes several days to induce a state of ketosis, so it takes some time before the body gets used to the normal carbohydrate metabolism. This is an area that still needs specific research.

## The Refilling of Carbohydrates

Usually, with a normal diet, muscle glycogen stores are always full. Under normal circumstances, an average person has about 350 grams. The consumption of these carbohydrates through diet and training followed by intake of many carbohydrates can duplicate this amount. During a normal diet, training has the ability to push up insulin sensitivity of the body which pushes up a muscle's capability to get insulin in the receptors. However, this push up in insulin sensitivity happens only in a well-trained body. This push up in sensitivity seems to occur as a result of glycogen consumption in the stronger muscles. Moreover, following a low carb regiment promotes the activity of the enzymes responsible for the accumulation of glycogen in the muscles.

So, if we put all the pieces together, we see that a carbohydrate-free diet, combined with a workout that runs out of glycogen stores, followed by a high carbohydrate diet promotes super-compensation of glycogen. It must also be said that a complete super-compensation of the muscles can take 3 or 4 days, even if most of the glycogen is stored in the first 24 hours. It can be said that the muscles are able to store 9 grams up to a maximum of 16 grams of carbohydrates per kg of lean mass.

For every gram of carbohydrates stored in the muscles, if you drink enough, another 4 grams of water will be retained in the muscles. As already mentioned, an average person (65 kg of lean mass) who follows a normal diet will have about 350 g of glycogen in the muscles. Since every gram of sugar holds 4 grams of water, it follows that it will also have 1 liter of water kept in the cells. With a super compensation at 12 grams, it is possible in theory, to store 1040 g of carbohydrates, which in turn, will retain 4160 g of water. This is an increase of about 3 times. Recent research shows that protein anabolism is also stimulated by the degree of cellular hydration. So, this super compensation would send an anabolic signal to the cells.

**Are there any side effects?**

The main one is fatigue, especially during the first week. One study even showed a decline in mental performance during the first week. However, this disappears as the diet is followed.

One of the most frequently asked questions is what effect this diet will have on the lipid profile of the blood. As you follow a low-calorie regimen, all ingested fats will be used as energy, and in addition to that, body fat will also be consumed. Healthy people will find an improvement in cholesterol values. Like any diet that causes drastic changes, it would be appropriate to do a blood test before starting and one after a few weeks.

Since it is a diet that almost completely eliminates carbohydrates, it also causes nutritional deficiencies. Therefore, it is essential that people who undergo this diet must take a good multivitamin and multimineral supplement. In addition, it is also essential to take a good fiber supplement.

Since the diet is high in fats, there is a greater production of free radicals, and therefore, it is not bad to make use of antioxidant supplements as well.

## Who should not follow the ketogenic diet?

The ketogenic diet is certainly excellent for increasing your health and energy level. Nonetheless, not everyone can follow this diet. If you fall within one of these categories that I am about to mention, I recommend that you do not follow the ketogenic diet for safety reasons.

**Pregnant women**. In this state, the body needs nutrients that derive from different sources. So, drastically restricting the sources of starches may have a negative impact on your child's health.

**Women who are breastfeeding.** During this stage, women need oxaloacetate, an essential compound to create lactose for breast milk, which is essential for the baby's growth.

**Athletes ready to begin a new season**. Athletes could get huge benefits from producing energy through ketones, but it can take 4 to 6 weeks before your body reaches ketosis. During this time, since your body has not yet gotten used to consuming fats as a source of energy, this can prevent you from achieving your optimal performance. To get the most out of a keto diet, give your body the time to adapt itself.

**People who have had their gallbladder removed**. Your gallbladder has the task of storing waste, giving your digestive system the ability to absorb the fat sources in the appropriate manner. Without the gallbladder, the fat sources are not absorbed in the right way. This can lead to nutritional deficiency. Why does this happen? It happens because most of the calories in this type of food come from fats.

**People who have had kidney problems**. If you have kidney issues in the past, the ketogenic diet could push up your chances of having kidney stones again. This is because the ketones increase the production of uric acid. On the other hand, if you have never had them, kidney stones can be prevented with a ketogenic diet because it increases the consumption of potassium thanks to the vegetables. Keeping yourself hydrated during the day helps decrease your chances of getting them again.

**People still in their growing phase**. This is because the ketogenic diet reduces the production of an essential hormone in the development of the bones and muscles of children and young adults.

Try typing "ketogenic diet" in a Google search. You will find more than 500,000 results linked to many sites, which are more or less reliable, and which explain how useful the diet is when used to lose weight quickly. Do you know the secret of the diet? The ketogenic diet eliminates sugars and carbohydrates.

There are those who propose the "paleo" version, inspired by the diet of primitive men. But is the ketogenic diet really so simple and affordable for everyone? Not exactly. To clarify is a document prepared by the experts of the American Association of Dietetics and Clinical Nutrition (ADI), based on the review of the most recent clinical studies conducted on the subject.

The ketogenic diet is based on the reduction or complete elimination of sugars from food for a short period of time. In search of alternative sources of energy, the body begins to burn fat, processing in the liver the substances called "ketone bodies" such as beta-hydroxybutyrate, acetoacetic acid, and acetone. Acetone is a transient metabolic disorder that in children can be caused by a feverish episode or prolonged fasting, an example of a "natural" ketogenic diet.

The production of ketones is indeed a sort of emergency plan, which serves to supply new fuel to the brain when it finishes the reserves of glucose.

The ketogenic diet can be considered as a medicine, and therefore, should not be done alone at home without the supervision of a doctor. Because of its physiological action at the central nervous system, it is recommended in cases of drug-resistant epilepsy. Some specialists also suggest it for the treatment of the most severe headaches, while new studies are evaluating its possible application in the field of neurodegenerative diseases like Parkinson's and Alzheimer's.

The ADI experts also remember its use in severe cases of obesity or refractory obesity, for example, in patients who must quickly lose weight to undergo surgery or to prepare for bariatric surgery. Moderate ketosis can also offer benefits in the case of type 2 diabetes, metabolic syndrome, and fatty liver (non-alcoholic fatty liver disease, NAFLD).

The ketogenic diet is contraindicated in pregnant and lactating women, in people suffering from hepatic, cardiac, or renal insufficiency, in young people with type 1 diabetes, in subjects with mental and behavioral disorders (anorexia, alcohol, and drug abuse), and in those who suffer from unstable angina, arrhythmias, porphyria, or have recently had a heart attack.

The ketogenic diet requires well-established goals and deadlines right from the start. It is usually carried out in cycles of three or four weeks, although some clinical trials have gone up to 12 weeks as well. The desirable weight loss is about 1-2 kilos a week, with peaks of up to 2.5 kilograms at the beginning. Please keep in mind that the scope of every diet should be to become healthier, not necessarily lose weight.

The diet should be modulated and customized according to the needs of the individual patient. In general, 30 to 50 grams of carbohydrates per day can be taken (less than 1 gram per pound of reasonable body weight), reaching the maximum level in males and large-sized individuals. The recommended protein intake is about 1 gram per pound of body weight per day, and the lipid level between 15 and 30 grams per day. The total kilocalories must be from 600 to 800 per day (to which are added to the kilocalories produced by the synthesis of ketone bodies, which are high in energy content).

If you use natural foods or whole foods, the diet may be a bit "limited and repetitive." For this reason, there are meals and substitute foods prepared only for particular occasions. ADI experts recommend a gradual diet, starting from more markedly hypocaloric and high protein, modifying in the next steps the protein intake (gradually reducing them) and the calories (to be increased just as gradually), with 3 to 4 phases each lasting an average of two weeks.

## What problems can you have?

Headache is the most frequent early side effect. Present in about a third of patients, it tends to disappear spontaneously within 72 hours. Subsequently, halitosis has been reported in the past (many patients report the need to use oral sprays or chewing gum, strictly without sources of carbohydrates), xerostomia (dry mouth), and constipation. Some patients also complain of reduced cold tolerance and postural vertigo.

For some time, there has been a total inversion with regard to the principles of weight loss and the basics of muscular anabolism.

# Classic Approach

## Food-induced Thermogenesis

The fundamentals of "traditional" dietetics suggest losing weight by exploiting also the specific dynamic action of food (ADS), or energy expenditure attributed to digestive, absorption, and metabolic processes.

In practice, with the same calories introduced in increasing the division of meals, it is possible to burn more energy to process them. This allows you to reduce the amount of time "on an empty stomach" avoiding the "hunger" and keeping the metabolism speedy.

## Cortisol and Thyroid Hormones

Some argue that this practice also favors the containment of an unwanted hormone, cortisol (also called "stress hormone") and maintenance of thyroid function (TSH and T3). Obviously, this system works as long as the caloric amount, the nutritional distribution, and the glycemic load-gauges of the meals are appropriate.

## Preventing Catabolism

At the same time, in the context of muscle growth, it is (or was) a common opinion that to promote anabolism, it was necessary to "feed" continuously (and "as much as possible," avoiding the increase of fat) muscle fibre cells in order to cancel any form of catabolism and promote photosynthesis, especially thanks to the insulin stimulus.

# Chapter 3: Three Keys to your Health

The ketogenic diet is essentially based on three principles.

1. *Reduction of simple and complex carbohydrates.*
   Foods containing carbohydrates must be eliminated,
   even though this is practically impossible. The portions
   of vegetables, which contain fructose are maintained,
   determining the percentage collapse of complex
   carbohydrates in favor of the simple ones, which are
   very low in quantity. These nutrients are the primary
   fuel of the organism and when reducing them "to a
   minimum," the body is forced to dispose of excess fat
   reserves. Moreover, carbohydrates are nutrients that
   significantly stimulate insulin (anabolic and fattening
   hormone), so that their moderation should also have an
   important metabolic significance.

2. *Quantitative and percentage increase of fats and only
   a minimal percentage of proteins keep the calorie-
   intake constant.* After eliminating carbohydrates,
   portions of the protein foods should be kept constant,
   increasing in parallel only the quantities of foods with a
   high content of fats (oils, oil seeds, oily fleshy fruits,
   etc.). In theory, this compensates for the caloric
   reduction of glucose thanks to the greater quantity of
   lipids. In practice, it is necessary to increase the portion
   and frequency of consumption of protein sources. Some
   justify this "correction" by stating that more proteins
   are useful for conserving lean mass. However, it should
   be specified that many amino acids are glucogenic (they

are converted into glucose by neoglucogenesis) and have a metabolic action similar to sources of carbohydrates, partially negating the effect on lipolytic enzymes and on the production of ketone bodies (see below). Moreover, in clinical practice, with the "hand calculator," the menu of the ketogenic diet is never normocaloric and provides less energy than necessary. So much so that, before venturing into such a strict regimen, you should try a well-balanced calorie diet.

3. *Production of ketone bodies.* The hepatic neoglucogenesis necessary to synthesize glucose (starting from certain amino acids and glycerol) is not fast enough to cover the daily glucose request of the body. At the same time, fat oxidation (closely related and dependent on glycolysis) "jams" causes the accumulation of intermediate molecules called ketone bodies. These ketones, which at physiological concentrations are easily disposable, in the ketogenic diet, can reach levels that are toxic for the tissues. Toxic does not necessarily mean poisonous, but rather "that causes intoxication." This effect is clearly distinguishable by the reduction of appetite, that is, the anorectic effect on the brain, although, like the heart, the nervous tissue is also partially able to use the ketone bodies for energetic purposes.

A healthy organism can function with high blood quantities of ketone bodies as well, whose excess is eliminated (we do not know how much effort is required by the body to accomplish this) from the renal filtration. Obviously, people suffering from certain pathologies (defect of insulin secretion, typical of type 1 diabetes, renal failure, also triggered by advanced type 2 diabetes, liver failure, etc.) have a very high risk of evolving in metabolic ketoacidosis, risking coma or, in some cases, even death.

# Chapter 4: How to Lose Weight in 10 Days with the Keto Diet

Ten days. How can you lose more than one or two kilos? That dress will not be enlarged by magic. It's time to get serious! This chapter contains all the information you need, ranging from calculating caloric needs, physical exercise, and ways to trick the brain and be able to feel satisfied by eating less. Only 240 hours left at the finish line, it starts now and there is one secret: ketogenic diet!

Determine your goals. How many pounds do you want to lose? Two? Five? To lose weight healthily, you should not lose more than 1/2 kilos a week, but during the first seven days, you can lose many more (mainly liquids), so do not be afraid to see your dreams broken for now. Simply decide how many pounds you would like to eliminate in the next 240 hours.
Suppose you want to lose 2.5 kilos. In practice, you will have to lose half a kilo every two days. As a pound is 3,500 calories, you will have to eliminate 1,750 calories every day.

Determine your needs. Let's continue with the current example. To lose one pound of weight a day, you have to create a daily deficit of 1,750 calories. It is worth pointing out that this is an ambitious goal, but we will nevertheless take it into consideration. Here's what you need to do to achieve it.

The first step is to calculate your basal metabolic rate (MB) and your daily caloric needs.

At this point, subtract 1.750 from the number of calories you should take daily. The result will set your daily maximum threshold. Obviously, the more you exercise the more calories you can eat.

Keep a food diary. You're serious, aren't you? Then take a notebook or download an application on your smartphone (there are many you can get for free) and start recording everything you eat. By putting the list of all the foods and drinks you eat every day, it will be much easier to understand where you went wrong. In the same way, it will be easier to bring out the progress! Moreover, the numerous possibilities offered by the many applications will help you stay motivated.

Your diary will allow you to track and count calories. In this way, if one day you cannot do any, maybe let yourself go a bit the next day and vice versa.

Plan physical activity. If you wanted to change your lifestyle over the long term, the idea of having to plan exercise for the rest of your life might seem too intense, but since you want to change your habits only for the next ten days, it is essential to do some concrete plans. The goal is to evaluate your commitments in advance and set up your training sessions at times that you are sure to respect. This way, you will not be able to make excuses!

It is advisable to exercise almost every day. An hour is excellent, but even 30 minutes can be enough to see results. If you need to split your training into one or two shorter sessions, it's not a problem. But if you think you do not have enough time to train, that is another story. You have to find it! There is always time for health, just wake up a little earlier or get to sleep a bit later.

Follow a ketogenic diet. You have a program to follow and you are motivated to achieve the goal, now, what you need to do is to make it happen. It might seem like a drastic move, maybe even a little respectful of your wallet, but go to the kitchen now and throw all the junk food and all the packaged foods that will not help you lose weight. If you are serious about losing weight, it is a sacrifice you must make. This is the only way to avoid falling into temptation.

Maybe you're thinking it's easier said than done. Your family members could oppose. In this case, it will be necessary to reach a compromise. For example, you could ask them to hide food or keep it in a place you cannot easily reach. Make sure they promise not to give in to your requests!

Understand how to eat a healthy keto diet. We come immediately to the point that you only have ten days. It is, therefore, essential to start eating right away. Having eaten for a lifetime, you might be convinced that you know how to feed in the right way. Unfortunately, when your mother taught you how to cook, she did not plan to help you lose weight. Here's how you should eat in an attempt to lose weight:

- Eat often. We are not talking about making six small meals a day as some diets recommend, but to separate the three main meals with two snacks. Making six small meals a day means forcing the body to constantly produce insulin without ever making it feel totally satisfied. Add two snacks between the main meals (during which you will have to try not to binge). They will help you eat less.
- Eat slowly. Chew your food. Put the fork down between each bite. When you eat quickly, your body does not

have time to tell you that you have reached satiety. As a result, it allows you to ingest a lot more food than you should. You have to give it time to record what you eat.

- Eat in small quantities. You will create an optical illusion. Generally, your brain pushes you to finish everything in front of you. Using smaller dishes, you will automatically eat less.

- Eat without doing anything else. When you stuff your food in a distracted way in front of the fridge, your mind does not register it as part of a meal. Sit down, concentrate, and pay attention exclusively to the consistency and taste of the food. Only afterward will you be able to return to your thousand daily commitments.

Blue is a natural hunger inhibitor. Nothing is better than a small blue plate resting on a blue tablecloth. To be on the safe side, you can also wear a blue shirt. No wonder restaurants use this color.

Use the caloric cycle strategy. Some studies have recently shown that taking up more calories than usual from time to time can favor a greater loss of unwanted pounds. Isn't it really good news? The reason is that by limiting the meals regularly, you force the body to slow down the metabolism and to assimilate to the last nutrient in order to stay healthy. By allowing yourself a "free" day from time to time, you allow the body to relax, speed up the metabolic processes, and eliminate accumulated fat in the form of stocks. During the ten days of the diet, consider scheduling a day or two to take some extra calories.

Try also the "carbs cycling". It is an alternative to the caloric cycle strategy based on alternating carbohydrate quantities. If you eat non-starchy vegetables and proteins (known to have a reduced carbohydrate content), it may be useful to plan a day when you consume a lot more carbohydrates. When it comes to burning them to produce energy, the body prefers them to fats and proteins. By including them in the diet, you will, therefore, strengthen the processes, thus favoring the desired weight loss.

Take it easy. Another aspect to keep in mind is the amount of stress. The more you are stressed the more you produce cortisol, a substance that causes you to eat. Tensions and worries induce problems such as "emotional eating", sleep disorders and less self-awareness. So relax, your waistline needs it.

Meditation or yoga is a good place to start. Yoga also allows you to burn calories. You will take two birds with one stone. At worst, find at least 15 minutes every day to sit in a quiet place and practice Zen meditation. Too many days end without you being able to find some time for yourself!

Sleep well. It is an advice given by science. It seems that the people who sleep the most are also those who weigh less. It is a sensible marriage. When you feel good, your body works well. Besides, you have less time to eat! So, commit yourself to sleep at least 8 hours per night. You will feel much better!

Leptin and ghrelin are the two hormones responsible for the mechanisms that regulate appetite and a sense of satiety. When their levels are not correct, the body is convinced of being hungry, while in reality, it is only tired. What's more, when you're sleepy, you tend to feel like eating sweets, to be attracted by the idea of eating outside the house, and ignoring the gym, the three bitter enemies of your desire to lose weight.

Be cautious of fast diets. It is obvious that spending the next ten days drinking only lemonade would allow you to lose several pounds. In a week, you would still feel like a rag and take up all the lost weight as soon as you start eating again. In addition, your metabolism would be ransacked. This is not a valid long-term solution! However, if what you want is to try a particular dress, try it, but be very careful and do not advise anyone to do the same.

Whether you want to rely on the benefits promised by eating only cabbage or maple syrup for a week, from spending entire days in the sauna or from a colon cleanse, you will find all the information you need and much more.

Keep this word in mind: water. It is the thing that comes closest to a miracle. When you drink a lot of water, wonderful things start to happen. Here is a list of benefits that should convince you to always keep a bottle of water at your reach.

- It satisfies you. The more water you drink, the less you want to eat solid food.
- It keeps your mouth busy. The more often you drink water, the less frequently you eat something else.
- Promotes the expulsion of toxins (and regular bowel movements).
- It is good for the skin and hair.

- Maintains healthy and hydrated muscles and organs.

Do not be afraid of veggies. In this case, the metaphor of the green light is very useful. If you want to lose weight and want to do it quickly, the most effective method is to eat lots of green vegetables. All vegetables are good for health, the green ones more than others. Known to be "nutrient dense", green vegetables contain only very few calories per serving, have a high satiating power, and are rich in vitamins and minerals, so they are perfect to help you achieve your goal.

All leafy vegetables are almost fantastic like cabbage, broccoli, spinach, lettuce, and even Brussels sprouts. You can eat them in large quantities without running out of the number of calories you have available daily.

Beware of white color. Unlike when you meet a traffic light, you must stop in front of white and not red. Foods of this color are often carbohydrates that have undergone an industrial refining process. This means that most of the fibers and nutrients have been eliminated during the processing. During the ten days of the diet, white rice, bread and pasta, and even white potatoes should be consumed only rarely or completely avoided.

To be precise, the human body needs carbohydrates, even during a ketogenic diet. Those contained in vegetables and whole grains are the ideal and healthier choice for the body as they are complex and not refined. Those industrially refined (simple carbohydrates) are rich in sugar, and should, therefore, be avoided.

You've probably heard of the Atkins diet (no carbohydrates). For a period of only ten days, it could prove to be effective, but it is nevertheless comparable to a lightning diet, so be prepared to have to suffer the consequences once finished. In conclusion, you can decide to avoid carbohydrates if you can, but with the awareness that there may be long-term consequences.

Say "Yes" to lean proteins. Your diet should consist of at least 10% protein. If you want to lose weight, it may be useful to consume even more. Protein favors muscle development and has a high satiating power: both of these factors help you lose weight. The advice is, therefore, to eat abundant quantities of fish, white meats, legumes, and soy (and its derivatives).

It is such a popular choice that some trendy diets recommend eating up to 30% lean protein every day. Some studies have found that combined with an exercise routine, a very rich protein diet can help reduce fats in the blood. In addition, proteins are known for their ability to limit blood glucose peaks, thereby, decreasing hunger. In this case, as well, the advantage is two-fold!

Learn to know good fats. This is an important skill as the body needs healthy fats. Eliminating them completely from the diet is not at all a good idea. The important thing is to know how to distinguish the good ones, unsaturated, from those harmful to health, "saturated". Those that are good for the body are contained in foods such as avocado, extra virgin olive oil, nuts, oily fish (such as trout and salmon), and in low-fat dairy products. In fact, consuming these healthy fats (naturally in moderate amounts) can help you lower your cholesterol levels and reduce your risk of developing heart disease.

Humans need to follow a diet consisting of at least 10% fat. Up to 25% can be considered a healthy quantity, but saturated fats should never exceed 7%. The latter, contained in red meats, eggs, poultry skin, and high-fat dairy products, are in fact considered harmful to health.

Since the egg is a useful source of protein at the same time, it is allowed to eat up to one a day. The important thing is not to exceed the quantities!

Reduce sodium consumption. In addition to blocking the blood vessels, forcing the heart to overwork, sodium causes the body to retain fluids. The widening of the waistline is a direct consequence of water retention. If you do not want to do it for the health of the heart, at least do to change the size of the pants!

A teaspoon of salt contains 2,300 mg of sodium. The daily requirement of our body is however only 200 mg. Since it is very difficult to stay within this limit, experts have raised it up to a maximum of 1,500 mg per day. In any case, it is important to never exceed 2,300 mg!

Avoid late night snacks. This rule is more psychological than scientific. During the night, human beings tend to eat wrongly and in a bad way. Promise to yourself not to eat anything after eight o'clock in the evening and keep faith to the commitment. If you feel hungry during the night, drink a large glass of water while keeping in mind what your goal is to lose weight. At the moment it might seem like a tough and not very "social" choice, but the next day, you'll be glad you stick to your keto plan.

This could be the most difficult part. Your friends go out in the evening, there are alcohol and snacks, and the thing you most want in the world is to be there with them. Make the following evaluations. You could go, but only if you are sure of being able to resist temptations, or you could give up, knowing that it is a sacrifice limited to a period of ten days. You will see that time will fly!

Lose weight by combining cardio activity with weight training. This is how it works. Cardio training allows you to burn calories faster than strength training. However, only a combination of both makes it possible to achieve the best possible results. There is nothing better for the body than to train all muscle groups in different ways. The cardio and weight activities have this effect, so find the time for both!

In these ten days, try to do cardio activity almost every day. The weights will instead be used on alternate days. If you want to intensify your strength training, concentrate daily on different muscle groups. The body needs a day off to recover.

Take every chance of moving the body. Going to the gym every day is an excellent choice, only a few people manage to keep such a pace. However, if you really want to get the most out of these ten days of the diet, the best thing to do is to take advantage of every other opportunity that keeps you active. Did you know that people who tend to constantly move nervously are more likely to be thin? Welcoming every possibility of making movement means reducing weight.

Try interval training. Cardio activity is useful, but recent studies have shown that interval training is even more effective when associated with a ketogenic diet. It also allows you to train in a more practical and quick way. Instead of running for 30 minutes, try to make quick sprints of 30 seconds each, separated by periods of recovery at a milder intensity (in which for example walk). Repeat for 15 to 20 times. This method allows you to burn a greater number of calories. Moreover, it maintains the rhythm of the heartbeat longer, thus allowing the body to continue to dispose of fat reserves even after the end of training.

Interval training offers several options in addition to running. For example, you can use the bicycle and alternate periods when you pedal intensely to short recovery phases.

Did the idea of continuing to burn fat and calories even after the end of training intrigued you? The effect is called "extra post-exercise oxygen consumption". When you push the body at a pace that it cannot sustain, it takes time for oxygen consumption to fall back into normal values. This is why you continue to burn more calories even while you are still.

Try "cross-training." Developing a workout routine is as easy as getting tired of it. The muscles, the mind, or both lose all stimulation and, when it happens, you start burning fewer calories because you stop working hard. The solution is cross training which gives you the opportunity to change the duration or intensity of the exercise or even move on to something completely new. Your body and mind will be grateful to you.

Light up your enthusiasm with new fun activities. Instead of the usual workout at the gym, sign up for a kickboxing class, go to the pool, or go hiking in the mountains. Invite a few friends to play basketball, tennis, or volleyball. In this way, you will be able to burn lots of calories without even noticing the effort.

Note when you get the best results. Probably, bodybuilding enthusiasts will tell you to first do the weights and then cardio activities. In contrast, cardio exercise advocates will force you to train strength only at the end. Still, others will tell you to train only in the morning on an empty stomach. What can be learned by this is that everyone gets the most out of what is best for him. Whatever it is that can make you feel upbeat even if it is to train in the middle of the night after having a snack!

Experiment! Perhaps you are convinced that you hate running because you only ran once after work. You may find that you like running early in the morning and lets you feel full of energy throughout the day. In these ten days, do several tests. You could develop a new passion that you will want to carry on for a lifetime.

# Chapter 5: How to Specifically Lose Belly Fat with the Ketogenic Diet

Fat in the abdominal area is associated with many disorders and diseases such as cardiovascular disease, diabetes, and cancer. Specifically, it is the deepest layer of the belly fat that puts health at risk. This is because "visceral" fat cells actually produce hormones and other substances. There are many dangerous and ineffective ploys to lose it. Although there is no certain infallible remedy for belly fat, this article describes the cause of the increase in waist size and what to do to eliminate it.

You have breakfast. Eating when you are trying to lose weight may seem a contradiction, but some studies have found that eating breakfast within an hour after you wake up keeps insulin levels stable and reduces LDL cholesterol (the "bad").

Take it easy. The research states that the secretion of cortisol (the hormone produced by the body when you're stressed) is associated with an increase in abdominal fat. Here's what you can do to combat the emotional tension of each day.

- Most people need at least 7 hours of sleep each night. Stop using electronic devices such as a computer and tablet half an hour before going to sleep to ensure a better quality of sleep.
- Take some time to relax. Even if you only have 15 minutes for lunch, find a moment to simply close your eyes, take deep breaths, and forget all your worries.

- Remove from the environment where you sleep everything that causes stress, as far as possible. Separate the space in which you sleep from the working space. Make sure you leave your worries behind as soon as you enter the room.

Plan to walk 10,000 steps a day. Research has found that visceral fat (abdominal) has increased by 7% after only two weeks in men who have reduced the passages from about 10,000 to less than 1,500 (without changing the diet).

- Try to walk to get to places that are within a reasonable distance. If possible, go to work, to school, or to the grocery store on foot.
- Get a pedometer and try to increase the number of steps every day.
- Take the stairs instead of taking the elevator and walk instead of using the car.
- Get up and do 30 steps every half hour. If you do a sedentary job, consider using a desk for standing work or those with a treadmill.

Give up refined cereals and eat only whole grains. A scientific study showed that people who ate only whole grains (in addition to five portions of fruit and vegetables, three of dairy products, and two of lean meat such as fish or poultry) lost more fat on their stomach than another group that had followed the same diet, but ate the refined cereals.

Whole grains are rich in fibers, which make you feel full for a long time and help you eat less, thus helping you lose weight.

Avoid refined cereals. For example, he eats wholemeal bread instead of white bread, which has undergone excessive processing and opts for wholemeal rice instead of shined rice.

Drink a lot of water. Some studies suggest that drinking water regularly during the day helps to speed up the metabolism regardless of the diet you follow. Drinking more water also helps the body to expel waste/toxins and improve overall health.

- Make sure to drink 250 ml of water eight times a day for a total of about two liters.
- Always carry a bottle of water with you so you can drink whenever you are thirsty.

Try to understand when you are not hydrated enough. You can be sure that you are drinking properly when the urine is light yellow or almost transparent. If it's darker than a post-it note, you have to drink more.

Significantly reduce the consumption of alcohol, sweetened beverages (such as sweetened teas, fruit-flavored, fruit punch, fruit punch, Coca-Cola, 7-Up, and Pepsi) and carbonated beverages.

Exercise following the HIIT principles. Research has found that interval exercise - an alternation of short, intense phases in which lots of energy are burned - can improve muscle endurance and development more quickly than standard training.

Avoid crunches at the start. Crunches and sit-ups allow you to strengthen your muscles, but it is unlikely that you will be able to see them under visceral fat. Actually, when you want to strengthen the abdominal muscles, the belly area may appear larger than it actually is. Your task now is to strengthen your back muscles to improve posture and bring your tummy back.

Do cardio activities. Perform aerobic exercises that help the heart to pump intensely, allow you to burn calories quickly, and facilitate fat loss throughout the body including the belly.

Remember that it is not possible to burn localized fats, but abdominal fat is generally the one that is lost first when training, regardless of the shape or size of the body.

Time the race time. Track your progress by noting the time you spend a mile. As your cardiovascular resistance improves, you may find that you run faster.

Relieves periostitis. If you suffer from a painful periostitis (you feel pain in the front of the shin when you run), maybe you have an overpronation (you tend to support most of the weight on the outside of the foot). In this case, you can wear specific footwear to reduce this discomfort.

Do not overdo it. Start with three cardio workouts a week or alternate this form of exercise with other lighter ones, such as walking for half an hour a day. If you ask your body daily too much, do not allow it time to recover and regenerate muscle mass with the risk of suffering some injury.

Add some resistance training to your routine. A study conducted in 2006 and published in an American journal specialized in sports and nutrition found that combining cardiovascular (aerobic) activity with resistance exercises is a more effective method than cardio exercise alone to get rid of abdominal fat. You can do resistance activities with dumbbells, weight machines, or resistance bands, as well as training on an unstable base to increase muscle activity.

Reduce the intake of calories and follow the ketogenic diet principles. Without control of the calories taken, you cannot lose visceral fat. Write down how much energy each day you help with a program you can find on the internet doing other online research and record everything you eat.
Remember that a 3,500 calorie deficit allows you to lose half a pound of fat. This means you have to burn 3,500 calories with exercise or eat 3,500 calories less each week than what you consume on a regular basis. Divide this information to know how many calories you have to renounce on a daily basis. To burn 3,500 a week, you must set a deficit of 500 a day. For example, you can do physical activity to burn 250 and reduce it with food.

Make sure you lose a pound a week at most. A greater weight loss can damage health and trigger a cycle of drastic diet, which leads to quickly regain lost weight.

Keep a food diary. Most people tend to underestimate what they eat. Make an honest assessment of your eating habits by writing down everything you consume for a week. Use an online calorie calculator to know the approximate number of those you introduce into the body. Starting from this point, find what you can give up.

Try a diet that includes 2,200 calories for men or 2,000 for women. In this way, a deficit should suffice to lose 0.5-1 kg per week depending on your level of activity. Some women need less energy, like 1800 or 1500 per day. Start with a contribution of 2,000 calories and reduce it further if you notice no results.

Do not fall below the minimum limit of 1200 calories per day, as it can result in serious damages for the body.

Eat some good fats. Studies suggest that a diet with a high ratio of mono-unsaturated fats, such as those found in olive oil, avocados, nuts, seeds, chocolate, and soybeans, can prevent the accumulation of visceral fat.

Trans fats (such as those found in some kinds of margarine and biscuits or in all products that contain partially hydrogenated oils) appear to increase abdominal fat deposits. Try to avoid them as much as possible.

Incorporate more fibers into your food. Soluble ones (found in apples, oats, or cherries) reduce insulin concentration, thus accelerating the loss of belly fat. Women should consume 25 grams per day, while the daily dosage for men is 30 grams.

Slowly integrate the fibers. If you currently eat only 10 grams per day, do not abruptly switch to 35 grams daily. The bacterial flora of the digestive tract needs time to adapt to new eating habits.

Eat the peel of fruit and vegetables. By increasing the portions of vegetable products, you can take a greater dose of fiber, but only if you also consume the peel that is its richest part. Do not peel the apples before enjoying them!

Cook peeled potatoes (both baked and pureed). If you decide to remove it, turn it into a healthy snack. Sprinkle with olive oil, rosemary, salt, and garlic before baking at 200°C for 15 minutes. Eating potato peelings take more vitamins and minerals than what you can get from the pulp alone (just remember to discard the green portions).

Eat more pea soup. These vegetables are a "superfood" regarding the fibers. A portion of about 180 grams contains 16 grams.

**Measure Progress**

Calculate the ratio between the waist circumference and the hip circumference. This value is a good indicator to know if you need to lose abdominal fat. Here's how to proceed:

1. Wrap a tape measure around the thinnest part of your waist, at the navel, and note the number.
2. Do the same by bringing the tape measure around the widest point of the hips, in the area where you can feel the bone protrusion about 1/3 from the upper portion of the pelvis. In this case, too, note the value.
3. Divide the circumference of the waist by that of the hips.
4. Know if it is a healthy value. Women should have a ratio no higher than 0.8 and men no higher than 0.9.

Keep measuring this data as you progress. After practicing the tips described in this chapter, continue measuring your hip and waist circumference to see if you're getting better.

The way the body distributes the adipose tissue is not at all under your control and depends on many factors including genetics, menopause, and so on. What you can "pinch" is the general amount of fat. If you keep a small percentage, it is not very important where it is, since it is still little.

Weigh yourself every day at the same time. Since body weight fluctuates according to the phases of the day, after a meal or after an intense movement, try to make the measurement a standardized process by always taking it at the same time.

Among the foods that we should put on the table in our keto diet, there are undoubtedly fresh and dried fruit, vegetables, whole grains (better if gluten-free but never always refined), legumes, and healthy condiments such as extra-virgin olive oil. Among animal proteins, if you really cannot do without it, it is better to prefer fish.

Vegetables are a great source of carbs and proteins, with a very low caloric index. This means that you can consume a large number of greens, while still losing weight due to a caloric deficit. Some of the best vegetables to eat in the ketogenic diet are the following:

• Artichokes

• Garlic

• Grapefruit

- Rocket salad

- Spinach

- Avocado

- Apples

- Broccoli

- Lemon

- Turmeric

As we have already said in the previous chapters, the duration of a diet varies according to the needs of the person following it. You can, in some cases, choose to follow a diet of this kind, obviously well-structured and with the right amount of food in each category (carbohydrates, proteins, and healthy fats), even in the short term. However, research has shown that it is advisable to stick to the ketogenic diet for longer periods of time to see the best results.

# Chapter 6: 15 Keto Recipes and the Importance of Having a Meal Plan

**We are increasingly talking about "Meal Prep" in America.**

Explaining what "Meal Prep" is very simple. The word itself gives us a precise idea: preparing meals ahead of time. Our lives are getting increasingly busier, cooking takes time, and it is easy to rely on gastronomy and pre-prepared meals. Meal Prep makes up for the problem because it is essentially "cooking in advance." There are different phases in meal planning. Here they are.

**First Phase: Meal Planning**
Personally, I have been doing "Meal Prep" for a couple of years now and everything starts on Saturday. I organize lunches, dinners, and snacks to know exactly how my menu will be structured during the week.

Meal planning means avoiding waste and following a more balanced diet that is compatible with my lifestyle. In general, my menu is structured in this way:

- Deadlines - What do I have in the fridge and freezer that is better to eat first? From this, I try to determine what I can prepare.

- Meatless Monday - On Monday, I follow a vegetarian diet (Meatless Monday is a good idea.)
- More protein - On Wednesdays, I have a gym session, so I go for protein and complex carbohydrates.
- Do not forget the fish - Friday is the fish day.

Once I have compiled my weekly menu, I can go shopping and then it's time for the Meal Prep.

## Second Phase: Meal Prep

Sunday is the day I cook most of the meals for the week. I prepare everything I can in advance. Vegetables cooked in the fridge last all week. Chicken is good up to 5-6 days as well as other types of meat.

Not everything, of course, can be prepared beforehand. After a few weeks, you will learn what you can prepare beforehand and what it is better to cook at the moment.

## The Benefits of Meal Prep

Let's look at some advantages of meal planning.

1. There are considerable savings.

Avoiding food waste by studying a menu is obviously a saving in terms of money and time. Cooking at home means you are able to avoid gastronomy, rotisserie, pizzerias, and bars. This is a direct saving. Home-prepared food comes at a lower cost.

Here in New York, a simple sandwich at a local bar can cost up to $5, which is $25 a week. I prefer to spend this money for a dinner at a good restaurant.

Moreover, my expense is studied and organized according to what's on my menu. This means saving a lot of money because I avoid compulsive purchases and saving a lot of time because I know exactly what I have to buy.

2.  You know what's in your food.

When you order a dish at the restaurant, you are not sure what you are ordering. You only have an idea of how the dish was made, but you do not know in detail the list of ingredients, nor the quality or quantity of the same. To be clear: what kind of oil did they use to fry your cutlet? And with what vinegar did they season your salad? How many calories does your salad really contain?

Preparing meals at home means having total control over what you eat. This means that you can prepare something you know you really like and that it is healthy for you. In particular, the ketogenic diet is much easier to follow when you are preparing your meals on time.

3.  You know exactly what you eat.

I try to eat as healthy as possible, and therefore, I try to eat a large quantity of fruit and vegetables, to be careful not to swallow too many sugars or saturated fats, to give space to fibers and proteins in my diet as well as foods that contain iron. Meal prepping allows me to eat much better. Therefore, my weekly menu, as you will find in the next chapter, includes snacks as well.

4. Other miscellaneous benefits:

- Flexibility - The freezer is your friend! Almost everything can be frozen, so you should not give up on unexpected dinner invitations.
- Right for everyone - Meal prepping is good for those like me who live alone or for large families!
- Additional time saving - Cooking once or twice a week means a lot less.

Now that we have covered the importance of a meal plan, let's take a look at some keto recipes.

## 1. Ketogenic Pancakes

*Ingredients:*
1. 10 gr of butter
2. 3 eggs
3. 50 gr of sugar
4. 100 gr of milk
5. 200 gr of flour
6. jam
7. 1 package of baking powder
8. Nutella or jam

*Preparation:*
1. Melt the butter and let it cool.
2. Divide the yolks from the whites.
3. Beat the egg whites until stiff and gradually add the sugar.
4. Beat the egg yolks with a whisk, adding the milk and

butter.

5. Mix the flour together with the baking powder, sieve everything, and mix it a little at a time with the mixture of egg yolks, butter, and milk.

6. When the flour is finished, add the beaten egg whites until stiff and mix gently to avoid disassembling everything.

7. Use the mixture immediately so that it does not lose its softness.

8. Heat a nonstick plate together with a knob of butter. Pass it lightly with a sheet of kitchen paper to absorb excess butter.

9. Keeping the heat of the pan not too high, pour 1 ladle at a time of freshly prepared mixture.

10. As soon as bubbles appear on the surface, turn the pancakes with a fork. As they are ready, place them on top of each other on a plate and keep them warm.

Pancakes can be spread with Nutella or jam, but traditionally, they are eaten hot with plenty of Canadian maple syrup.

## 2. Ketogenic Meatballs

*Ingredients for 4 servings:*
- 500 g of ground beef
- 1 whole egg
- 20 g of Parmesan cheese
- 20 g of breadcrumbs
- 1 clove of garlic
- 1/2 glass of white wine
- 100 g of carrots
- 1 tablespoon of fennel seeds
- 1 tablespoon of dried parsley
- Salt to taste
- 3 tablespoons of extra virgin olive oil

*Preparation*

- Let the lean butcher grind your lean meat, then season it with salt, the clove of garlic cut into small pieces, breadcrumbs, grated cheese, beaten egg, and herbs.
- Mix everything well with your hands and if necessary, adjust the consistency of the dough with the breadcrumbs if it is still not very compact. Shape the meatballs the size of a walnut.
- Wash, clean, and slice the carrots on wheels, then heat the oil in a sufficiently large skillet and sauté the carrots and the meatballs over high heat, blending with white wine.
- Let it evaporate for a few minutes, stirring well. Stir the pan by the handle to avoid breaking the meatballs.
- Cover and cook over low heat for about 15-20 minutes, stirring occasionally to cook the meatballs on all sides. Serve the meatballs hot.

## 3. Spicy scrambled eggs

*Ingredients for 2 servings*
- 4 medium eggs
- 50 g of tuna in oil
- 1 teaspoon of mustard
- a pinch of pepper
- a pinch of salt
- chives and oregano
- 2 teaspoons of extra virgin olive oil
- 10 gr of mustard
- aromatic herbs (the ones you like the most)

*Preparation*

1. Place the eggs in a saucepan with water, cover, and boil for 15 minutes.
2. Allow the eggs to cool and peel them.
3. Cut them in half, take 3 egg yolks out of 4 and place them in a small bowl. Drain the tuna well from the oil.
4. Mash the yolks with the tuna with a fork, add the mustard, pepper, salt, and aromatic herbs. Once you have a smooth mixture, fill the egg whites.
5. Serve and season the eggs with oil and a sprinkling of pepper and herbs.
6. If you do not like the taste of mustard, you can replace it with curry powder or turmeric.

## 4. Ketogenic Biscuits

*Ingredients for 10 servings*

- 80 g chickpea flour
- 90 g coconut flour (from pulp)
- 30 ml extra virgin olive oil
- 1 whole egg
- 1 tablespoon of honey
- 50 ml of coconut milk
- lemon peels
- 1 pinch of salt
- 2 teaspoons of ginger
- 1 sachet of baking powder

*Preparation*

1. Put the coconut flour, the chickpea flour, the pinch of salt, the ginger powder, and the sachet of yeast in a bowl. Mix well with a wooden spoon.
2. Grate the peel of an untreated lemon and add it to the flour.
3. Beat the egg with a whisk and add the honey first, then the oil and finally the milk, continuing to whisk with a whisk.
4. Combine the liquid ingredients with the flour and knead it well until you get a smooth ball. Rest for half an hour.
5. Obtain 2-3 cm diameter balls from the dough and lay them in an oven-lined lacquer. Crush them with your hands to get the shape of biscuits.
6. Bake for 20-30 minutes at 170 ° C.

## 5. Vegetable passion

*Ingredients*
- 10 gr of butter
- 45 gr of pumpkin
- a tablespoon of oil
- curry
- a pinch of salt
- a pinch of pepper
- 1 egg
- a pinch of walnut nutmeg
- 50 gr of parmesan
- 

*Preparation*

1. You will need a small round baking dish (they are called ramekin); choose it high enough so that butter does not come out during the cooking process. To mix the ingredients, a small bowl is required and can be useful.
2. If you want to prepare several flans together to freeze them, you have to multiply all the ingredients and every single flan (for 3 flans, 3 times 45 grams of pumpkin and not 135 grams of pumpkin).
3. Weigh separately all the ingredients. For the egg, mix thoroughly the yolk and light it with a whisk or a blender. Use a pumpkin that does not have too much water in it, such as Hokkaido (small, crushed, with dark green peel) or, better still, butternut (small with elongated neck).
4. Heat the oven to 180 degrees. Cut the pumpkin into strips not too thin and put it on one pan with oven paper underneath. Spray it with a spray (this oil is not weighed, with the spray, it will still be much less than

one gram); spray over the curry (also unweighted, not exaggerated), salt and bake for 5 minutes in the ventilated oven.

5. Grease the ramekin (the bottom and the sides) well, with all the butter in the recipe. In a bowl, stir the egg, cream, and almond flour. Add a pinch of walnut nutmeg. Pull out the pumpkin and let it cool for two minutes. Pour the mixture into the ramekin and add the pumpkin.

6. At this point, cover everything with grated Parmesan, spreading it in a uniformed manner (help yourself with a spatula). Bake for 25-30 minutes in the oven at 180° (ventilated). Bake until there is one beautiful crust on the surface. It's not like a soufflé, so when you get it out of the oven, it will not deflate. Serve directly in the ramekin, it will remain warmer.

## 6. Keto Curry

*Ingredients*
- 10 gr of butter
- a tablespoon of olive oil
- 2 onions
- 1 package of curry
- 2 thyme leaves
- parsley
- fresh vegetables of your choice
- 100 gr of chicken
- 100 gr of rice

*Preparation*
1. To make the curry veal stew, heat the butter with oil in

a pan and brown the chopped onions. When they have become transparent, add the pieces of floured meat and brown them well over high heat, turning them often because they take color evenly. After about five minutes, add salt and pepper. In the meantime, melt the curry powder in a large glass of hot water.

2. Pour over the meat the curry dissolved in water, mix very well and cook covered, over medium-low heat for about an hour. Stir occasionally, and if the meat should dry out too much, add a little hot water.

3. When cooked, add the thyme leaves and the minced parsley. Transfer to the serving dish and serve the curry veal stew accompanied with pilaf rice or plain boiled rice.

# 7. Ketogenic Pasta

*Ingredients*
- 150 gr of spaghetti
- 1 lemon
- 10 gr of butter
- a pinch of salt
- 100 gr of ricotta

*Preparation*
1. To prepare spaghetti with lemon, place a pot with plenty of slightly salted water on the stove. As soon as it boils, cook the spaghetti according to the package directions.
2. In a pan, melt the butter, add the lemon, and stir for two minutes, then add the juice.
3. In a separate pan, toast the pine nuts, taking care that they do not burn, then wash and dry the basil.
4. Drain the pasta, keeping a glass of cooking water, add it to the lemon juice and mix well until it is all blended.
5. Add the Ricotta and a ladle of cooking water and mix well until it has formed a velvety cream that wraps the spaghetti.

## 8. Eggs and Tuna

*Ingredients for 2 servings*

- 4 medium eggs
- 50 g of tuna in oil
- 1 teaspoon of mustard
- a pinch of pepper
- a pinch of salt
- chives and oregano as you like
- 2 teaspoons of extra virgin olive oil
- other aromatic herbs (the ones you like)

*Preparation*

1. Place the eggs in a saucepan with water until covering and boiling for 15 minutes.
2. Allow the eggs to cool and peel them. Cut them in half, take 3 egg yolks out of 4 and place them in a small bowl. Drain the tuna well from the oil.
3. Mash the yolks with the tuna with a fork, add the mustard, pepper, salt, and aromatic herbs. Once you have a smooth mixture, fill the egg whites.
4. Serve and season the eggs with oil and a sprinkling of pepper and herbs.
5. If you do not like the taste of mustard, you can replace it with curry powder or turmeric.

## 9. Autumn Tastes

*Ingredients*

- 100 gr of pork chop
- 1 pumpkin
- 10 gr of butter
- a tablespoon of olive oil
- a pinch of pepper
- a pinch of salt
- a tablespoon of soy sauce
- 25 gr of the cheese you like the most
- 2 potatoes
- 2 onions
- mixed vegetables

*Preparation*

1. To prepare the pork chops with pumpkin cream and cheese, first prepare the vegetable pieces, which will be used to prepare the pumpkin cream.
2. Then, prepare the pumpkin cream. Cut the pumpkin into slices, remove the outer peel, remove the seeds, then reduce the pulp first to strips and then into cubes. Peel the potatoes and cut into cubes too. Then take the onion, clean it, and chop it finely. Transfer it to a pan with the oil and sauté over a gentle heat.
3. Once the onion has reached the browning state, add the pumpkin in the pan together with the potatoes. Slowly add a few ladles of vegetable stock to cover the vegetables.
4. Season with salt and pepper and cook over low heat for 25-30 minutes, adding some vegetable stock

occasionally. Once the vegetables are cooked, turn off the heat and start blending them with an immersion mixer until a smooth and homogeneous cream is obtained. Add a sprinkling of nutmeg and cinnamon and mix together. At this point, your pumpkin cream is ready, so put it aside.

5. Take the chops and beat them with the meat until they are about 1 cm thick, then chop the sage and rosemary and place them in a non-stick pan with a little oil.

6. Put the chops in the pan, season with salt and pepper and leave to brown on both sides, turning them from time to time with a pincer so that they cook on both sides.

7. Once cooked, remove them from the pot and keep them warm. In the same pot in which they cooked the chops, pour the previously prepared pumpkin cream, add the soy sauce and mix well.

8. Add the chops, season with the pumpkin cream, then cut the cheese into slices and place one above each chop. Cook for 1-2 minutes to melt the cheese, sprinkle everything with thyme leaves. Mix well and your pork chops with pumpkin cream and cheese are ready to be served!

## 9. Taste of the Sea

*Ingredients*
- 1 monkfish fillet
- pink pepper
- a pinch of salt
- a tablespoon of olive oil
- 200 gr of puff pastry
- 1 lemon
- 1 package of saffron
- mixed vegetables

*Preparation*
1. To prepare the monkfish in saffron and lemon sauce started with the cleaning of the monkfish fillet. Cut into slices; with a knife remove the bones inside and then remove the skin. Cut the clean slices in half and make some tiny parts, tying them all around with the kitchen string. You need to prepare 8 monkfish medallions.
2. Remove the leaves from the thyme sprigs and place them on each nibble, then put the fish aside. Now, prepare the sauce. In a pan, pour oil and lemon. Add the saffron bag and let it melt.
3. Add the pink pepper and thicken the sauce as well. Then, sift the rice flour into the pan and mix well with a whisk to thicken the flour without creating lumps. Continuing with the whisk, pour the vegetable pieces as well. Season it with salt and pepper and cook for a few minutes until the sauce becomes creamy.
4. Once ready, turn off the heat and set it aside. In another pan, heat the oil and add the garlic. Once golden, remove the garlic and place the monkfish medallions.
5. Cook for a few minutes at medium heat and gently turn the tidbits with a kitchen tongs. When they have taken a

nice brown color on both sides, turn off the heat. On a serving dish, pour the saffron and lemon sauce (which will be the base on which to lay the fish) and place the monkfish medallions on it. Finish by pouring a few drops of sauce on the portions obtained and served.

## 11. Chicken and avocado

### Ingredients

- 1 avocado
- ½ lemon
- 60 gr of oil
- salt
- parsley
- 100 gr of chicken
- 1 ginger

### Preparation

1. For the recipe of chicken and avocado salad with ginger sauce, fry the chicken meat and pick it up in a bowl.
2. Peel the ginger and grate it, then squeeze the pulp in your hands, and pour the juice into a small bowl. Add the juice of 1/2 lemon, 60 grams of oil, a pinch of salt, and parsley, and blend with a dipping mixer to obtain a sauce.
3. Clean the avocado and cut into chunks. Season the chicken with the ginger sauce and complete with avocado chunks.
4. To make it taste better, you can also add the peeled lemon.

# 12. Cocoa And Mint – A Keto Dessert

*Ingredients*
- 100 gr of butter
- 50 gr of coconut
- coconut oil
- peppermint extract
- cocoa powder

*Preparation*

1. Combine 100 grams of melted coconut butter, 50 grams of grated coconut, 1 tablespoon of coconut oil, and half a teaspoon of peppermint extract.
2. Mix well and pour into cream puffs or muffin molds, filling them halfway.
3. Put in the fridge to harden (about 15 minutes).
4. Mix 2 tablespoons of melted coconut oil and 2 tablespoons of cocoa powder.
5. Remove the peppermint mixture from the refrigerator and pour the cocoa mixture into each mold over the peppermint.
6. Refrigerate until the bombs harden.
7. Before serving, remove the bombs from the refrigerator and let them rest for about 5 minutes.

## 13. Rice and Vegetables

*Ingredients for 4 people*
- 300 gr parboiled rice
- 160 gr tuna in drained oil
- 200 gr mozzarella cherries
- 120 gr pitted black olives
- 80 gr pesto
- extra virgin olive oil
- a pinch of salt
- 2 fresh basil leafs

*Preparation*

1) Boil in salted water 280 gr of parboiled rice, drained, and seasoned with 80 gr of pesto and a little extra virgin olive oil, mix well and let it cool.
2) Add 120 gr black pitted olives, 200 g of cherry-cut mozzarella cut in half, and finally, 160 g of drained tuna and crumbled.
3) Sprinkle with a ground of pepper and mix well to flavor the rice.
4) Place the rice salad in the dishes, garnish it with some basil leaves and serve. If you want a more elegant presentation, grease a ring mold, pour the seasoned rice, crush a little surface to fill all the holes well, and before serving, let stand for at least 10 minutes.
5) Turn the mold onto a serving dish, remove the mold, and decorate with the basil leaves.

## 14. Ketogenic Brioche

*Ingredients*
- 10 gr of butter
- 100 gr of flour
- 1 package of baking powder
- 50 gr of milk
- a pinch of sugar
- a pinch of salt

*Preparation*
1. Melt the butter and let it cool. Pour the flour into a bowl. Add the baking powder, sugar, and salt.
2. Stir, and then incorporate the eggs, the melted butter, and finally the milk.
3. Stir quickly with a fork, cover with the food foil and leave to rise for 3 hours at room temperature, in a warm place, and away from drafts.
4. After this time, transfer the dough in the refrigerator and let it rest for 24 hours.
5. Before baking the brioche, leave it at room temperature for a couple of hours. Turn on the oven at 180°C. Transfer the dough into a 23 cm long plum cake mold with butter and flour.
6. Brush the surface with milk and decorate with the granulated sugar. Cook in the hot oven for about 40 minutes.

## 15. Ricotta Explosion

*Ingredients*
- 150 gr of pasta
- 50 gr of ricotta
- Parmesan 30 gr
- a tablespoon of oil
- a pinch of salt
- a pinch of pepper

*Preparation*

1. To prepare this recipe called "pasta and ricotta", first boil a pot of salt water and cook the pasta for 10 minutes or the time reported on the package.
2. In the meantime, you can prepare the dressing: using a spatula, sieve the ricotta in a bowl through a strainer with a tight mesh to obtain a nice smooth consistency.
3. Then, add the grated Parmesan and fresh cream and mix well with the spatula. Add the thyme leaves, stir again, and finally add salt and pepper.
4. Drain the pasta, keeping some of its cooking water, and pour it directly into the bowl with the ricotta mixture.
5. Mix well the pasta with the sauce, lengthening it with a ladle of cooking water, if necessary. Your creamy pasta and ricotta are ready to be served!

## Ketogenic Water

If you are looking for an alternative to water that is non-alcoholic but refreshing and healthy, flavored ketogenic waters are the right choice. They are beautiful to look at, good to drink, and help you to hydrate and purify yourself because they are prepared with natural ingredients like vegetables, fruits, and vegetables. Plus, since they do not contain sugar or other sweeteners, they are calorie-free and help you detox from the first sip.

## When to drink flavored water

You can drink keto water always and without limits: during the day to cool off, for lunch or dinner instead of water or as an alternative to tea and other drinks when you're out with friends. The advantage is that being free of caffeine and rich in fruit, they are a perfect drink to offer both to adults and children.

## What you need to prepare keto waters

The main ingredients are water, mineral, or even tap if it is the one you usually use.
Then, seasonal fruit and vegetables, to be cut and left to infuse together with the aromatic herbs or spices you love. Before starting, prepare a glass bottle or carafe to be filled and stored in the fridge and leave the keto water to infuse for a period of 1 to 12 hours. The flavored water should be consumed within a few hours after filtering it.

## 1. Keto Water - Pineapple, Lime, and Pineapple Sage

It is among the most purifying keto waters, thanks to the pineapple and lime that encourage diuresis and help you to eliminate toxins.

Ingredients for 1 lt. of water:

1 slice of pineapple.
1 lime.
1 tuft of pineapple sage.

## 2. Keto Water - Cucumber, Fennel, and Chives

In addition to the above-mentioned benefits, keto water can also be deflating, like this one, which is prepared with fennel and cucumber, is useful for getting a flat stomach.

Ingredients for 1 lt. of water:

half a cucumber.
The tips and external parts of fennel.
1 tuft of chives or mint.

## 3. Keto Water – Melon, Apple and Mint

The keto waters are tasty as well as healthy, and this one with melon, green apple, and mint is good, very fragrant, and very also suitable for children.

Ingredients for 1 lt. of water:

1 slice of melon (a clove)
half green apple (from organic farming)
1 tuft of mint

## 4. Flavored Water - Peach, Kiwi, and Lemon Balm

Keto and relaxation: with peach and kiwi, you can purify yourself. With the lemon balm, you relax and abandon the tensions of the day from the body and mind.

Ingredients for 1 lt. of water:

1 Peach
1 kiwi
1 tuft of lemon balm

## 5. Keto Water - Celery and Radish

The keto water can be flavored even with vegetables. The result is a less appetizing taste, but very useful for your body shape.

Ingredients for 1 lt. of water:

1 celery coast with leaves
4 small or 2 medium / large radishes

# Chapter 7: A Conceptual Discussion about Food

Have you ever wondered why we eat? It is one of those simple questions behind our discovery of the complex mechanisms that run our lives. The first reason behind "why we eat" is that it allows us to grow from being an infant until we reach our maturity as an adult. The second function of nutrition is to conserve life. Food gives energy to our body and maintains a caloric level sufficient to conserve the temperature of the body of each species. In this case, human beings have a normal body temperature of 37 degrees Celsius.

What happens if the food is not consumed? The body takes calories from the fat tissue, which is temporarily stored mostly in your belly when you eat. Good health refers to keeping the process of food intake and food expenditure in balance. If you eat too much, you go beyond the natural purpose for which fat deposits exist. This will make you obese.

In the richest countries, obesity is an increasingly widespread phenomenon. Various explanations are given as to why there is widespread obesity in such countries. For some, the impulse to eat beyond measure comes from an ancestral hunger, like if it is a sort of command left in their brain and ready to be activated in the presence of food.

For others, the explanation is psychological. In fact, we create an abnormal situation with this almost neurotic need for excessive nutrition. Just look at how many mothers overfeed their children today.

A positive food education has been lost.

Today, everything is turned upside down, and it is often the children who threatened their parents not to eat if they do not turn up the television or condescend to their desires. Instead, the golden rule is to eat just enough, as we have seen in previous chapters. Not only because of the cardiovascular risks related to overweight, but also because more food is introduced, and more risks are incurred for cancer. The risk of cancer is proportional to the amount of food that is introduced: more food, more risks.

We will certainly be against the current trends, but those who follow the ketogenic diet believe that many food pathologies are linked to a culture that has lost sight of what really is necessary to survive. Bad diseases such as anorexia and bulimia did not exist almost 30-40 years ago when there was a good education in food and attention to its good use. Think about how they managed to remain healthy despite having a poor economy at that time. As Bismarck said, you can get out of the rules of healthy eating on your birthday, but you do not have to celebrate your birthday every day.

Man is a primate which means that he is a modified monkey, and the monkey has maintained very basic metabolic characteristics. Primates have been and still are vegetarians and also interact with the plant world because they basically eat only fruit.

The flowers, from which the fruit came from, are colorful and fragrant because they have to attract pollinating insects that allow fertilization. The fruits, equally colorful and fragrant, attract animals including humans. However, this harmony and this synergy between different kingdoms and worlds at some point in human history started to suffer from a great problem: the great glaciations. The plants disappeared almost completely. Many vegetarian animals perished miserably.

The human species was saved, and from a vegetarian species became a carnivore one. The turning point of human nutrition was the ice that covered the planet. Men became carnivorous, but also maintained the metabolism of a vegetarian primate. In short, our organism is programmed for the consumption of fruit and vegetables, and to return largely to this type of food can only benefit us. This is why, in the ketogenic diet, it is advised to consume a lot of fresh green vegetables, as they are the primary source of the few carbs the diet allows.

# Conclusion

Thank you for making it to the end of this book, we really appreciate your interest in the ketogenic diet. Now, you have all the information that you will need to start changing your lifestyle and getting back in shape. It is always a pleasure to see our readers turn their health around after reading our books and we know you will be the next success story.

We would like to end this book by encouraging you to take the first step. We know, it is always the most difficult, but we also know that once you have done it, everything becomes easier. During the first days of the ketogenic diet, we suggest that you listen to your body more than ever. It will be amazing to see how it starts transforming using the new patterns you are offering it.

This is your time. This is the moment when your health begins a new journey. Stay consistent, stay motivated.

You got this!

CPSIA information can be obtained
at www.ICGtesting.com
Printed in the USA
LVHW051003251120
672557LV00004B/682